Aromatheraphy
for
Natural Health

Also by the Authors
Aromatherapy for Scentual Awareness
Aromatherapy for Lovers and Dreamers
Aromatherapy for Men
Aromatherapy for Meditation and Contemplation
Aromatherapy for Scents and Sensuality

Aromatheraphy
for
Natural Health

Judith White and Karen Downes

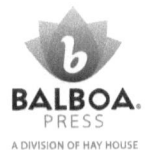

BALBOA.
PRESS
A DIVISION OF HAY HOUSE

Copyright © 1997, 2011 Judith White and Karen Downes

The moral right of the authors has been asserted.

Balboa Press books may be ordered through booksellers or by contacting:

Balboa Press
A Division of Hay House
1663 Liberty Drive
Bloomington, IN 47403
www.balboapress.com
1-(877) 407-4847

Because of the dynamic nature of the Internet, any web addresses or links contained in this book may have changed since publication and may no longer be valid. The views expressed in this work are solely those of the author and do not necessarily reflect the views of the publisher, and the publisher hereby disclaims any responsibility for them.

ISBN: 978-1-4525-0206-9 (sc)
ISBN: 978-1-4525-0210-6 (e)

Any people depicted in stock imagery provided by Thinkstock are models, and such images are being used for illustrative purposes only. Certain stock imagery © Thinkstock.

Printed in the United States of America

Balboa Press rev. date: 6/10/2011

Editing by Rachel Eldred

Text Photography by Elizabeth Dobbie

*We dedicate this book to all who
have journeyed with us
on our Aromatic adventures.*

Acknowledgements

Katerina Lettas for overseeing the project. A special thanks to our researcher and editor, Rachel Eldred, and the whole Nacson clan for never losing their sense of humour.

Contents

Introduction

HAVE YOU EVER HAD AN INCREDIBLE IDEA THAT YOU *HAD* TO ACT upon? Whenever you'd mention it to anyone, they'd say "yeah, what a great idea, I love it!" And then life gets in the way and you put your idea on the backburner, dabbling with it every now and again but never quite getting it done.

Aromatherapy For Natural Health was one of those ideas. We'd always wanted to compile a book where an A-Z of oils, ailments and complementary therapies could be found in one easily accessible guide. It would be a simple, easy-to-use guide, enabling the reader to quickly decide for him/herself an appropriate choice towards bringing greater balance into their lives. It would be a resource for the home that everyone could use. Now, at last, *Aromatherapy for Natural Health* has become a reality.

What makes this book particularly valuable is that we've explored the extensive world of Aromatic healing and also covered the wonderful world of complementary therapy. We believe that combining aromatherapy with an appropriate complementary therapy will make the best possible contribution towards optimum health.

When it comes to achieving optimum wellbeing, there are two universal laws that promise a healthy start: a well balanced diet and exercise. The "laws" governing good health are no great secrets. Even if we choose not to abide by these laws we are inherently aware of them. After a well balanced meal, or 30 minutes of moderate exercise, our whole being seems to lift and glow a healthy radiance. On the other hand, if we eat a less nutritious meal after sitting around in front of the television all day, our radiance seems to drop and we have less energy.

While exercise and a well balanced diet are important factors in a healthy lifestyle so too is adopting a positive attitude towards stress. Stress is a part of everyone's life and while some of us can't seem to live with it, we certainly can't live without it. A certain amount of stress in our lives enables us to achieve goals or initiate and fulfill dreams (we certainly wouldn't have completed this book if this weren't the case!). It's how we handle stress that is important. If we allow it to become too great, our health is compromised: many doctors today recognise a correlation between stress and ill health. The best way to handle stress is to listen carefully to that small voice within that's telling you exactly what it needs, ie learn to follow your intuition.

Throughout the ages, intuition was the primary force when it came to health care. Whenever an individual fell ill they would trust their own intuition, or that of a local healer, to let them know which berry to chew, or drink to brew, to promote healing.

Modern society now has the best of both worlds when it comes to health: medical science *and* Mother Nature's pharmacy. We do not trivialise the role medical science plays in our lives for it certainly has its place. Having said that we shouldn't ignore our own "inner knowing" when it comes to healing either. Optimum wellbeing incorporates a healthy balance between intuitive "knowing" and professional know-how.

Aromatherapy for Natural Health has been written to re-kindle this approach to healing, encouraging you to better understand the individual needs and wants of your body. When it comes to healing, allow your intuition to influence you toward making appropriate health care choices.

In ancient China, physicians and healers were hired only when their patients were well. If a patient fell ill, payment was withdrawn. Thus it was in the physician's best interest to ensure the patient's wellbeing.

If a physician observed that a patient was inappropriately dressed in cold weather, the patient would be advised to put some warmer clothes on and swallow a particular berry, known to assist in the prevention of colds and flu. This was an effective form of preventative medicine. Today, with a far greater understanding of the science of aromatherapy and other complementary therapies, we recommend you explore the possibilities presented by regular use of these efficacious treatments as valuable health insurance.

As you prevent the wheels falling off your car, or the roof of your home collapsing, so too should you prevent your health deteriorating. Neglect often has serious and long term ramifications.

Aromatherapy for Natural Health has been designed for easy reference. First, flick through the A-Z guide to ailments for general information about your particular concern then check with the A-Z of essential oils for information about the specific oils recommended. Following this you can refer again to the list of ailments to see how best to use each specific oil to assist healing. Finally, the complementary therapy chapter provides a summary of some of the most efficacious natural therapies available today. A list of conditions each natural therapy has shown to have a positive effect upon is also included. *(See back of book for Natural Therapy Associations and Societies.)*

We do not profess to be medical practitioners, or to have all the answers to every ailment. We strongly advise you to consult your chosen health practitioner on those occasions when you may not be 100 per cent confident about a diagnosis. In this way you can ensure that your self-diagnosis gets the benefit of a second opinion.

Here it is, your companion to wellbeing. If we had realised how much fun it would be and what fascinating insight it would offer, we may not have taken so long to bring the idea into fruition. But in the immortal words of John Lennon, "Life is what happens to you when you're busy making other plans."

CHAPTER ONE

THE AROMATIC WARDROBE

I

The Aromatic Wardrobe

THE POWER OF SMELL IS BEAUTIFULLY HIGHLIGHTED IN THE BOOK *Perfume* by Patrick Süskind. Readers are taken on a fascinating and poignant journey through one man's experience with the sense of smell: his sense is so acute that he can literally smell the essence of everything around him. So if he was to come and enjoy breakfast at your house, he'd be able to smell the coffee bubbling on the stove as well as the tart smell of lemon meringue pie you had baked in the oven two days previously. As well as these smells, he'd be able to identify your own special fragrance, too.

While Patrick Süskind may have imagined this story into creation, its sheer brilliance lies in its realism. After all, everything that exists in this world has an essence; this is what gives things their smell.

Some essences are strong, rose for example, others more subdued, like apples.

We are able to extract smells, or aromas, from the leaves, stems and flowers of plants, shrubs and herbs through their volatile oil. This and the fact that they are insoluble in water is what gives them their name, i.e. essential oils.

Essential oils differ from fragrant oils in that they are not chemically constituted by humans. Essential oils are the working tools of aromatherapy, and for aromatherapy to have therapeutic benefits you must be sure you are using Mother Nature's gifts; not human-made imitations.

With the use of essential oils, aromatherapy can have an effect on all the different systems of our body: skin, circulation, muscles and joints, respiratory system, digestive system, reproductive system and endocrine system. Most oils will have qualities that overlap with other oils, although no two oils are alike.

Essential oils enter our body via two routes: skin and breath. They then enter the blood, transporting the oils throughout the entire body so they can either support or instigate healing. That's the beauty of aromatherapy: it's a holistic therapy. It doesn't simply mask symptoms but encourages the body towards self-healing. For example, lavender will provide relief from the effects of eczema and it will also calm the body, giving it a better chance to heal itself.

Aromatherapy, although scientifically recognised, is a highly intuitive and intricate art. Care should always be taken when using essential oils: they should never be used undiluted over large areas of the body and they must avoid direct contact with eyes and mucous membrane, i.e. inside the nose. Because essential oils are not soluble in water, if irritation or allergic reaction occurs, remove oils immediately with a massage base oil or milk. As a cautionary note, too, do not use citrus oils *(Bergamot, Lemon, Orange, Lime, Mandarin or Grapefruit)* on the skin in the presence of ultraviolet light, i.e. sunbaking or sunbeds. When reading the essential oil compendium below, please note any contra-indications and cautions.

The descriptions of the oils below should be used in conjunction with Chapter Two. In this way, you'll be able to fully appreciate the benefits of aromatherapy.

B A S I L

Country of origin: Egypt
Botanical name: Ocimum basilicum

BASIL ASSISTS IN THE TREATMENT OF ALL KINDS OF RESPIRATORY ailments such as bronchitis. It provides temporary relief from headaches and colds and assists in the prevention of muscular cramps and spasms. Basil is also an excellent nerve tonic.

You can use Basil for concentration and decision making for it has a clarifying effect on the brain. Choose it if you're just about to conduct or attend a business conference, or for any environment where you are wanting the participants to be more focused when receiving important data that is to be remembered. If you're studying, call on Basil to assist you to focus your concentration.

Basil oil, pale yellow in colour, is distilled from the leaves/flowers of the Basil plant.

Caution: *Avoid topically during pregnancy.*

BERGAMOT

Country of origin: Italy
Botanical name: Citrus aurantium s. bergamia

BERGAMOT GIVES TEMPORARY RELIEF FROM THE SYMPTOMS OF eczema, cold sores and cystitis. It is a very uplifting oil and helps to disperse nervous anxiety or depression. As a massage oil it is excellent when treating acne and oily skin problems or dermatitis.

If you are a teacher, presenter or facilitator of information to an audience, simply breathe in the aromatic vapours to disperse pre-presentation jitters.

This delightfully fresh and citrus essential oil is made by pressing the rind of a fruit like a miniature orange. Bergamot is the distinct flavour found in Earl Grey Tea.

Caution: *Photosensitive: Do not use externally in the presence of ultra violet light ie: when sunbaking or using sun beds.*

BLACK PEPPER

Country of origin: India
Botanical name: Piper nigrum

USE BLACK PEPPER TO EASE AWAY MUSCULAR ACHES AND PAINS OR stiffness after physical exertion. This essential oil assists to strengthen poor muscle tone and revive the body from fatigue. It provides temporary relief from rheumatic pain and the symptoms of chilblains, and supports the digestive system.

An excellent oil to use for enhancing your self-image, building your self-esteem and instilling a greater sense of confidence. A great oil for when your patience is wearing thin and your energy levels are flagging.

C H A M O M I L E
(ROMAN & GERMAN)

Country of origin: Hungary and England
Botanical names: Anthemis nobilis (Roman)
and Matricaria chamomilla (German)

THESE TWO VARIETIES OF CHAMOMILE ARE SIMILAR. BECAUSE they affect both the body and mind, you can use them to treat inflammation.

Roman Chamomile is a particularly sweet fragrance compared to German Chamomile which is far more herbaceous. Roman Chamomile is effective when seeking relief from colic or any other gastric disturbances, pre-menstrual symptoms including cramps, or mouth ulcers. It also helps to relieve nervous tension, stress and mild anxiety.

German Chamomile has wonderful anti-inflammatory properties. It can be used in the treatment of skin allergies such as eczema or to ease the symptoms of red, inflamed skin. It also provides temporary relief from arthritis, laryngitis, tonsillitis and sinusitis. Use it to provide relief from the cough of bronchitis.

C A R D A M O N

Country of origin: Ecuador
Botanical name: Elleataria cardamomum

CARDAMON HELPS TO RELIEVE INDIGESTION AND FLATULENCE WHEN massaged into the abdominal area. Brings comfort to heartburn and colic, and helps to ease coughs and relieve the symptoms of catarrh.

It's great as an oil to remedy stress, providing relief to body and mind.

C E D A R W O O D

Country of origin: USA
Botanical name: Juniperus virginiana

CEDARWOOD USED IN A VAPORISER OR INHALED IS A GREAT HELP with chest complaints such as catarrh and bronchitis. Used in conjunction with Rosemary, it can assist in restoring hair growth and can retard thinning hair.

One of the oldest known essential oils, Cedarwood may be used to release chronic anxiety and reduce stress.

The fragrance of Cedarwood brings emotional support; you can call on Cedarwood to provide a more harmonious atmosphere to a tense situation.

C L A R Y   S A G E

Country of origin: Austria
Botanical name: Salvia sclarea

CLARY SAGE PROVIDES RELIEF FROM MENSTRUAL PAINS AND HELPS
to maintain a healthy digestive system. It is the most euphoric of all
essential oils and is particularly effective in providing relief from stress
and mild anxiety. Clary Sage relaxes and uplifts the most despondent
person and releases depressed thinking.

Distilled in the northern hemisphere from the Clary Sage flowers, it
has a sharp and slightly nutty aroma.

Caution: *Avoid topically during pregnancy.*

C Y P R E S S

Country of origin: Spain
Botanical name: Cypressus sempervirens

CYPRESS MAY HELP TO PREVENT ASTHMA ATTACKS. IT IS USEFUL IN treating conditions where excess fluid is a problem and provides relief from the discomfort of haemorrhoids and pre-menstrual tension. It also gives relief to a runny nose and helps to disperse nervous tension.

This highly astringent oil is distilled from the leaves and berries of the tree. Its woody fragrance is often used in men's toiletries.

EUCALYPTUS

Country of origin: Australia, China
Botanical name: Eucalyptus globulus

EUCALYPTUS IS AN EXCELLENT DECONGESTANT AND ITS ANTI-bacterial and anti-viral properties can help to stop the spread of infections. You can use it to relieve the pain and itching of chicken pox, shingles and cold sores. Some surgeons use Eucalyptus-impregnated gauze to cover wounds. Eucalyptus oil is the best-known protection against winter ills and can bring relief to arthritic pain.

Caution: *Avoid topically during pregnancy.*

F E N N E L

Country of origin: Spain
Botanical name: Foeniculum vulgare

Ideal as an alternative to Peppermint, Fennel aids the digestive system, providing relief from nausea, colic and flatulence, and is the ideal after-dinner 'mint'. It helps to relieve nervous tension, stress and mild anxiety.

The oil is distilled from the dried and crushed seeds of the Mediterranean plant Foeniculum vulgare which has a delicious aniseed aroma.

Caution: *Avoid topically during pregnancy. Avoid topically on hypersensitive or damaged skin.*

F R A N K I N C E N S E

Country of origin: East Africa
Botanical name: Boswellia thurifera

FRANKINCENSE HAS A REJUVENATING EFFECT AND IS ESPECIALLY good for mature skin. It assists in dispensing fear as it fortifies and comforts.

The effect of Frankincense on the mind and emotions is calming and it may be used to promote a quietening of the mind when meditating or to help unwind after an overwhelming day.

The resin from which Frankincense is distilled has been burnt on altars for centuries. Sourced now, as then, from Saudi Arabia and Somaliland, it has a penetrating, soothing aroma.

Caution: Do not apply to hypersensitive or damaged skin.

GERANIUM

Country of origin: Egypt
Botanical name: Pelaragonium graveolens

GERANIUM HAS USES IN SKIN CARE, PARTICULARLY WHEN THE SKIN is dry, as with dermatitis, eczema and severe cases of dandruff. It provides relief from pre-menstrual symptoms and is beneficial during times of stress and mild anxiety.

Geranium is a good balancer for mood swings or emotional highs and lows during those 'mid-life' experiences and through times of change. It has a calming and relaxing effect if you're feeling uptight.

The distilled leaves produce a typical 'flower' oil used regularly in the perfumery industry as a substitute for Rose. It originates mainly in North Africa.

Caution: *Not to be used topically on red and inflamed skin.*

GINGER

Country of origin: China
Botanical name: Zingiber officinalis

*W*HEREVER RIGIDITY OCCURS IN THE BODY, BE IT ARTHRITIS, muscular stiffness and tension or even in the case of poor circulation, this oil gets things moving. It helps to maintain a healthy digestive system and provides relief from the pain associated with cystitis. Ginger may help to relieve the symptoms of colds, too.

With its warming qualities, Ginger is a great booster of confidence. It energises and strengthens the body and the mind.

Caution: *Avoid topically during pregnancy.*

G R A P E F R U I T

Country of origin: Israel
Botanical name: Citrus paradisi, Macfaden

GRAPEFRUIT IS A VALUABLE OIL FOR PROTECTION AGAINST infectious diseases. Use it to energise and activate the body before exercise. Uplifting and refreshing, it alleviates stress and anxiety and promotes alertness, sharpening the senses for greater performance.

Caution: *Photosensitive. Do not use externally in the presence of ultraviolet light, ie: sunbaking or sunbeds.*

JASMINE ABSOLUTE

Country of origin: India
Botanical name: Jasminum officinale

JASMINE ABSOLUTE IS RENOWNED FOR ITS APHRODISIAC QUALITIES and ability to arouse physically and emotionally. It can be used to soften dry, irritated and sensitive skins. It is an extremely sensual extract which arouses and warms, restoring a deep sense of confidence and elevating self-esteem.

Jasmine Absolute is an excellent oil to bring balance and optimism, most helpful when choosing to release frigidity *(either emotional or physical)* or depression. It has also been used to alleviate nervous exhaustion.

J U N I P E R

Country of origin: Austria
Botanical name: Juniperus communis

JUNIPER CAN BE USED IN ASSISTING THE TREATMENT OF FLUID retention. It works on the emotions to rid the mind of 'waste', thereby relieving anxiety. As a purifier of the blood, it can be used to relieve the symptoms of arthritis, joint pain and gout. It also provides relief from the pain and burning sensation associated with cystitis.

The Chinese revere the Juniper tree for its immortal quality. The oil is distilled from its ripe berries and has a fresh aroma like turpentine. Juniper is an ingredient of gin and works to stimulate the appetite – hence the drink 'gin and tonic' as an aperitif.

L A V E N D E R

Country of origin: Bulgaria
Botanical name: Lavandula augustifolia, Lavandula officinalis

LAVENDER'S PROPERTIES RANGE FROM ANTI-BACTERIAL AND CELL stimulating to acting as a sedative and insect repellent. Probably the most popular and versatile essential oil, Lavender has a soothing and calming effect, balancing and normalising any given condition.

If you're feeling irritable, agitated, short tempered or find that you are taking everything personally, call on Lavender to soothe away frayed emotions. Wearing Lavender is nearly as nurturing as having a pair of loving arms draped around your neck and a soothing word whispered into your ear.

It's an excellent oil as a general tonic when you're recovering from an illness. It can be strengthening and nurturing, providing relief from sleeplessness, nervous tension, stress and mild anxiety.

L E M O N

Country of origin: Sicily
Botanical name: Citrus limonum

$\mathcal{L}$EMON OIL HELPS THE BODY DEFEND AGAINST INFECTION. USED neat in combination with Thyme essential oil, it can get rid of warts. It is useful for the treatment of oily skin. It provides temporary relief from stress and mild anxiety and helps to maintain a healthy digestive system.

When you want to stay wide awake and enlivened whilst reading, reviewing or studying, call on Lemon essential oil as it stimulates focus during study and relieves the mind from brain strain.

This essential oil is pressed from the outer rind of the fruit and has the familiar citrus aroma.

Caution: *Photosensitive: Do not use externally in the presence of ultraviolet light, ie: sunbaking or sunbeds.*

L E M O N G R A S S

Country of origin: India
Botanical name: Cymbopogon flexuosus

LEMONGRASS OIL IS TONIFYING AND CLEANSING FOR THE WHOLE body. It provides temporary relief from headaches, constipation and muscular aches and pains. It also helps to maintain a healthy digestive system. Lemongrass assists recovery from intense physical activity. It's a powerful tonic and has a stimulating effect on the whole system.

Caution: Avoid topically during pregnancy. Avoid topically on hypersensitive or damaged skin.

L I M E

Country of origin: Peru
Botanical name: Citrus aurantifolia

BY ACTIVELY WORKING ON CLEARING PHYSICAL AS WELL AS emotional issues, this oil is great for obesity, congestion and poor circulation. It helps to clear problem or blemished skin and provides temporary relief from muscular cramps and spasms and the symptoms of flu.

Lime, along with the rest of the citrus family, is refreshing and uplifting. This oil promotes clarity and assertiveness, making it an excellent choice if you're feeling doubt or confusion. Because of its stimulating effect on circulation, you can use *Lime* oil to induce warmth to cold hands and feet, or to move you into activity.

Caution: Do not use externally in the presence of ultraviolet light, ie: sunbaking or sunbeds.

M A N D A R I N

Country of origin: Sicily
Botanical name: Citrus reticulata

MANDARIN IS EXCELLENT FOR DIGESTIVE DISORDERS AND intestinal discomfort, especially when massaged into the abdominal area in a clockwise direction. It helps to move excess fluid in the body and activates the liver.

Mandarin's sweetness inspires and brings a sense of calm and tranquillity. This oil is a favourite for restlessness and insomnia as it soothes away anxiety and tension. It also provides temporary relief from menstrual cramps and muscular cramps and spasms.

Caution: Do not use externally in the presence of ultraviolet light, ie: sunbaking or sunbeds

MARJORAM

Country of origin: Egypt
Botanical name: Origanum marjorana

THE WARM, PENETRATING AROMA OF MARJORAM WORKS TO LESSEN both physical and emotional responses. Its comforting properties help those experiencing grief. It provides temporary relief from insomnia, pre-menstrual tension, muscular cramps and spasms, and headaches. It is excellent for hurt muscles and tension.

This is the oil to choose when your body and soul are crying out for deep relaxation. Marjoram, as an excellent sleep inducer, will help to rebalance the body's time clock' for shift workers.

Caution: *Avoid topically during pregnancy.*

M Y R R H

Country of origin: East Africa
Botanical name: Commiphora myrrha

THIS THICK, STICKY, REDDISH BROWN OIL HAS A PUNGENT AROMA and is a very good expectorant and astringent, helping with all kinds of coughs and colds. It can be used to heal mouth ulcers and in the treatment of gingivitis.

Myrrh is strengthening and rejuvenating, providing relief from the discomfort of haemorrhoids, flatulence and diarrhoea.

This rare oil is distilled from the resin of a small, thorny tree which grows in difficult countryside. Legend has it that Arab shepherds collected the resin from the beards of their goats.

N E R O L I

Country of origin: Tunisia
Botanical name: Citrus aurantium, amara

NEROLI MAKES YOU FEEL MORE SETTLED, ESPECIALLY IF YOU ARE tossing and turning prior to sleep. It calms hysterical behaviour and is an excellent vein tonic. If you have varicose veins or broken capillaries (red cheeks or nose is the visual display for broken capillaries) then use Neroli. Because Neroli assists new cell growth, it is useful in skin care, particularly for dry skin.

Neroli is especially helpful when you want to minimise anxiety; it can bring relief to all kinds of stressful situations. When you reduce stress and anxiety, you increase your sensual arousal.

This oil takes its name from an Italian princess who used it as her favourite perfume. Distilled from the flowers of the Seville orange, it has a beautiful perfume, particularly when diluted.

O R A N G E

Country of origin: Brazil
Botanical name: Citrus aurantium, sinensis

ORANGE RELIEVES THE RESTLESSNESS OF INSOMNIA, CREATING an opening for rest, and can help ease acute headaches. In skin care it is useful for cleansing oily skin. If you smoke, try using Orange to soften and release any congested pores. It provides temporary relief from stress and mild anxiety.

Distilled from the outer peel of oranges, this refreshing and uplifting oil blends well with others.

Caution: *Do not use externally in the presence of ultraviolet light, ie: sunbaking or sunbeds.*

PALMAROSA

Country of origin: India
Botanical name: Cymbopogon martini

USE PALMAROSA IN YOUR DAILY SKIN CARE REGIME TO PREVENT dryness. Use with Lavender to heal scar tissue. It can also be used for its antiseptic qualities to relieve the symptoms of colds and flu. With its ability to calm and strengthen, this oil is excellent for nervous exhaustion as it brings balance and restoration to frayed nerves. It provides temporary relief from sinusitis and from the cough that comes with bronchial irritation. It also provides relief from the pain and burning associated with cystitis.

P A T C H O U L I

Country of origin: Indonesia
Botanical name: Pogostemon cablin

*P*ATCHOULI WORKS WELL AS AN ANTISEPTIC TO HEAL CHAPPED OR broken skin and fungal infections including athlete's foot. Old scar tissue responds well to a blend of Patchouli and Lavender.

Patchouli provides temporary relief from the symptoms of eczema and the effects of psoriasis, and assists in treating diarrhoea.

This oil has a rich Eastern aroma which can relieve anxiety and depression and may even have an aphrodisiac quality, particularly when blended with Ylang Ylang. Patchouli really came into its own in the 1960s when it was used to promote love and peace.

P E P P E R M I N T

Country of origin: USA
Botanical name: Mentha piperita

THE CLASSIC STOMACH/DIGESTIVE REMEDY, PEPPERMINT HAS excellent anti-spasmodic properties and is a pleasant general stimulant. Inhaled directly from the bottle, it clears the head and is an effective treatment for travel sickness or sinus congestion.

As one of the stimulating essential oils, Peppermint promotes clear thinking, activates the brain and engages thoughts.

Caution: *Avoid topically during pregnancy. Those who suffer from epilepsy or convulsions should also avoid its use.*

PETITGRAIN

Country of origin: Paraguay
Botanical name: Citrus aurantium amara

PETITGRAIN IS A GREAT HAIR TONIC FOR OILY OR GREASY SCALPS. In the summer months especially, Petitgrain makes an excellent anti-perspirant. It helps maintain a healthy digestive system and provides temporary relief from sleeplessness, muscular aches and spasms, stress and mild anxiety.

Use Petitgrain as a tonic for the nervous system while recovering from any stress-related conditions. This oil brings an inner sense of strength and stability. With its fortifying qualities it encourages communication, expressiveness and openness.

P I N E

Country of origin: Siberia
Botanical name: Abies siberica

INHALATIONS OF PINE OIL ARE GOOD FOR RELIEVING CHEST COLDS and catarrh. It also has a stimulating effect on the circulation. This essential oil is particularly good for adults who suffer from asthma or as a tonic to the lungs of those who smoke. It can also be used as a liver tonic, aiding the maintenance of a healthy digestive system. It provides temporary relief from muscular aches and pains and bronchial cough.

Pine needles are firm and strong by nature. The Pine tree exudes strength and purpose and these are the qualities your body drinks in as you absorb the aromatic molecules.

Dry distillation of the needles, cones and young twigs collected in northern Europe and Russia produces a pale, fresh, resinous aroma.

Caution: *Avoid topically on hypersensitive or damaged skin.*

R O S E

Country of origin: Bulgaria
Botanical name: Rosa damascena

ROSE WORKS POWERFULLY ON YOUR BODY, ESPECIALLY ON THE reproductive system and it has a restorative effect on the liver *(especially after a generous drinking session)*. It is particularly valuable for use in skin care as a tonic.

Rose is the most potent healer of the essential oils. Just one drop is all you'll require for most purposes. The exquisite and powerful perfume works on the depths of your emotions, nurturing and restoring power and confidence. Cleopatra made Rose oil famous for its aphrodisiac qualities. She used it to seduce her lovers and negotiate trading terms with merchants.

One of the elite essential oils, it wears a price tag better regarded as a 'personal investment' as it takes thousands of rose petals from Bulgaria to make one drop of Rose.

ROSEMARY

Country of origin: Morocco
Botanical name: Rosmarinus officinalis

ROSEMARY HAS A STRONG EFFECT ON THE NERVOUS SYSTEM, acting as a brain stimulant to heighten sensory perception and memory. Traditionally used in hair care, mostly as a rinse or scalp rub, it can stimulate hair regrowth. It provides relief to muscular aches and pains, and assists in the treatment of constipation. It also provides temporary relief from headaches.

One of the earliest oils used, Rosemary essential oil is distilled in Tunisia, Yugoslavia, Spain and France.

Caution: Avoid topically during pregnancy. Those who suffer from epilepsy or convulsions should also avoid its use.

R O S E W O O D

Country of origin: Brazil
Botanical name: Aniba roseaodora

ROSEWOOD CARRIES ANTISEPTIC PROPERTIES WHICH PROMOTE THE body's own natural defence system, thereby assisting in fighting coughs, colds and winter chills. To emotionally rebalance and recharge, this oil carries a restorative quality, both emotionally and physically, and it elevates and uplifts even the most despondent mood.

This tropical evergreen tree with a reddish bark and heartwood is native to the Amazon region. Rosewood blends well with most oils, especially citrus, woods and florals.

S A G E

Country of origin: Albania
Botanical name: Salvia officinalis

Smelly feet and armpits surrender to Sage and it's deep-cleansing qualities help purify the dirtiest pores and skin. It helps in the treatment of fluid retention and is an effective liver tonic, assisting in maintaining a healthy digestive system. It can be used for the treatment of tinea and is beneficial during times of stress.

Valued throughout time as a sacred herb, it sources mainly from south-eastern Europe.

Caution: *Avoid topically during pregnancy. Those who suffer from epilepsy or convulsions should also avoid its use.*

S A N D A L W O O D

Country of origin: India -- Eastern District
Botanical name: Santalum album

*A*s a cosmetic ingredient, Sandalwood brings moisture to dry skin. It has been used most successfully to treat sore throats and laryngitis. It provides temporary relief from the pain and burning associated with cystitis. It relieves the discomfort of haemorrhoids and helps to maintain a healthy digestive function.

A strengthening aroma which releases irrational fears, Sandalwood can have a stabilising influence through many life changes. It is used to promote strength and courage especially for people undergoing a lot of changes.

The oil is distilled from the heartwood of the tree. Long used in India as a perfume and incense, Sandalwood seems to live up to its reputation as an aphrodisiac.

TEA TREE

Country of origin: Australia
Botanical name: Melaleuca alternifolia

TEA TREE OIL WORKS TO FIGHT AGAINST BACTERIA, VIRUSES AND funguses. If there was ever first aid in a bottle, this is it. If you have a mouth ulcer, boil, infected cut or abrasion, gum disorder, tinea, wart, wasp or bee sting, thrush, etc, Tea Tree is the oil to use.

It is also a powerful immune-stimulant which helps the body to respond by fighting invading organisms. This oil protects you when you wear it on your body. It has an energising effect on the body and mind, especially when used first thing in the morning.

Caution: *Avoid topically during pregnancy.*

T H Y M E

Country of origin: Spain
Botanical name: Thymus vulgaris

*I*F YOU LIKEN TEA TREE TO THE SOLDIER AGAINST BACTERIA, THEN it is appropriate to call Thyme the army. Thyme is a powerful force against long-term colds, flu or viruses that seem to persist. It acts as an antioxidant in the body and is said to prolong the degeneration of brain cells.

This is a potent oil and only the smallest amount——sometimes even half a drop, is all that is required to produce results.

It is an excellent oil for respiratory, mouth and throat infections (never use directly inside the mouth, on the vagina or on any mucous membrane, as this oil is very strong) and works to stimulate the production of white blood cells, strengthening the body's resistance to infection.

Its refreshing herbaceous fragrance blends well with Sandalwood.

Caution: *Avoid topically during pregnancy. Avoid topically on hypersensitive or damaged skin. (A mucous membrane irritant.)*

V E T I V E R

Country of origin: Java
Botanical name: Vetiveria zizanoides

VETIVER BRINGS STRENGTH TO THE DEEPER LAYERS OF THE SKIN and supports the body's ability to absorb nutrients. It is used successfully to alleviate stress and is a useful skin care aid for mature skin types.

A deeply relaxing oil, Vetiver comes from the root of the plant and is responsible for its nourishment. We therefore acknowledge the drawing power of Vetiver as the bearer of opportunities and possibilities.

YLANG YLANG

Country of origin: Comores (off the coast of North Africa)
Botanical name: Cananga odorata

Y LANG YLANG WILL BE EFFECTIVE IN YOUR SKIN CARE PROGRAM AS it has a balancing effect on both dry and oily skins. It will help regulate rapid heart beat and rapid breathing, and assists in the prevention of muscular cramps and spasms. It is a strongly exotic sensual oil that blends well with other floral, citrussy and woody oils.

An anti-depressant essence possessing sedative and aphrodisiac qualities, Ylang Ylang is mainly used for its calming and relaxing properties.

Ylang Ylang has the ability to arouse the senses. It has a provocative and alluring fragrance and is a tonic to the emotions of the heart, helping to disperse anger and frustration.

Originating in Indonesia, Ylang Ylang is used in perfumery and cosmetics. The powerful aroma is from the 'flower of flowers' and is identifiably heavy and sweet.

Caution: Not to be used topically on red and inflamed skin.

Massage Base Oils

Often essential oils are added to a massage base oil for massages and body rubs.

AVOCADO

A rich oil known for its high vitamin content. A 10 per cent addition can be added to any blend for a velvet-like consistency which will soften the skin.

JOJOBA

This rich body oil is a natural fluid wax, high in protein and minerals. As a wax, Jojoba should go solid when placed in a fridge or in extremely cold conditions. It is extremely nourishing for the skin and hair.

MACADAMIA

Extremely high in vitamin A, this true Australian oil with its warm nutty aroma assists rejuvenation. An excellent body oil for daily skin care to nourish and moisturise.

PEACH KERNEL

High in vitamin A, this carrier oil helps to maintain a healthy complexion. Moisturises and softens the skin for a wonderful body massage.

OLIVE

Rich in proteins and vitamins, this carrier oil brings warmth to the body during massage. This oil is particularly good during winter months. Warm slightly before applying to the skin for rapid absorption.

SWEET ALMOND

Rich in nutrients, this massage base oil is light in texture and will lubricate the skin for a wonderful massage. This is an excellent massage base oil as it allows your hands to easily glide over the body when giving a massage.

WHEATGERM

Extremely high in vitamin E, this carrier oil will help extend the life span of your blended aromatherapy oils. It assists as an antioxidant and will benefit any scarring on the skin. A 10 per cent addition to your massage base oil blended with your essential oils will help prevent oxidisation.

It's important to remember the following three points when using massage base oils.

- *The oils should always be cold pressed vegetable oils to maintain vitamins and minerals.*
- *Store in glass containers, preferably amber glass.*
- *Vegetable oils do turn rancid after a period of time and should be used within 6-8 months with the exception of Macadamia and Jojoba which last for several years.*

Proper Essential Oil Care
for Infants *and* Children

When treating children with essential oils, we have to employ a sliding scale of dosage to mirror their growth. Children respond brilliantly to essential oils and you should use them with confidence with all children––even babies––although some caution has to always be taken with the very young.

Pure essential oils are very powerful substances and you should always keep dosages low when working with children. Just 1 drop in their bath water or 1 drop diluted into 10ml of massage base oil when applying to the skin. Avoid contact with the face at all times and their hands, which they often use to rub their eyes. This applies to children under 5 years.

New-born babies are particularly sensitive, but diluted essential oils can work wonders to clear up any troubles your baby may have in the first 12 months of life.

The most effective ways to treat various common baby ailments involves Vaporisation and Massage, which allow the molecules of essential oils to be effectively embraced for their healing benefits.

Just place your vaporiser or a bowl of steaming water on the floor, well away from baby, and add the essential oil so that it rises with the vapours and permeates the atmosphere. Just 4 drops of essential oil into your vaporiser or to one litre of hot water is quite adequate for babies.

The following oils are the only essential oils we recommend for babies under 12 months. Each of them is to be used singularly and always diluted when applied to the body: Roman Chamomile, German Chamomile, Lavender, Sandalwood and Cedarwood.

These essential oils can be used as safe alternatives to pharmaceutical drugs in many cases of childhood illness. This is something you as a parent will have to prove to yourself, but we encourage you to have confidence in the oils and the aromatic treatment of your children.

CHAPTER TWO

METHODS OF USE

2

Methods of Use

YOU CAN EMPLOY THE HEALING ART OF AROMATHERAPY IN MANY delightful ways: essential oils are so versatile. Each method involves either direct contact with your skin or inhalation, in many cases both.

The skin is the body's largest organ. It protects against unwelcome guests and is intimately associated with our sense of touch. Most of us love the sensations aroused when we are delicately touched by a loved one. When we combine the healing forces of touch with the delightful aromas of essential oils our skin is nurtured and stimulated. After applying essential oils to the skin they penetrate the epidermis *(outer layer of the skin)*, travelling through the dermis *(lower layer)* where they enter the bloodstream to travel freely through the body. The oils will then be attracted to the areas of the body that they have an affinity with. Each oil in its natural chemical composition performs a healing action.

Essential oils can also be carried through the body via the lymphatic system. The lymph constitutes the major part of the body's immune system. The lymphatic system can be likened to a ship with a full crew. When essential oils enter the body, they board the ship as nutritional and medical supplies for the crew. They are a complete maintenance repair kit for the vessel itself.

The other route essential oils take to enter our bodies is via our breath, or smell. It's in this way that essential oils have an effect on our emotions. The aromas are inhaled, stimulating the olfactory receptors which are directly related to the brain's limbic system. *(The limbic system stores smells, moods and short and long-term memory.)* This explains the phenomenon of associating certain smells with people, places and emotions.

Essential oils are assimilated, digested and excreted. They leave the body predominantly by the breath, sweat glands and urine.

While inhalation and massage are the two main methods in which essential oils can be used, there are many derivations. Following is a detailed compilation of the different methods of essential oil use.

AROMATIC BATHING

In Western cultures, bathing is mainly associated with cleansing. In Aromatic bathing we have adopted the wisdom of the ancient Romans and the bathing rituals of the Japanese to create a bathing experience for replenishing the body, mind and spirit. Add 3-5 drops of essential oil to a full bath. Agitate the water to disperse the oil evenly before entering the water. To optimise the benefits of the essential oils, soak for 10 minutes, inhaling deeply. On completion gently pat your skin dry. One drop of essential oil in the bath water is appropriate for children 5 years and under.

Note: When using citrus oils, reduce this recommended dosage by half.

AROMATIC DRESSING

A daily ritual of applying essential oils to dress the largest organ of the body—the skin. Simply choose the most appropriate essential oils for the day to prepare your mind, body and emotions. This method was created to protect and nourish the skin as a preventative health care tool. With the application of essential oils, you are truly dressing from the inside out.

Into 10mls of massage base oil, eg sweet almond or jojoba, add 3-5 drops of essential oil in total. A selection of one, two or three essential oils can be blended. One drop of essential oil in 10ml of massage base oil is appropriate for children 5 years and younger.

AROMATIC MASSAGE

Aromatic massage enables you to surrender to a state of calm. Depending on the oils chosen, you can create a stimulating or sedating effect while moisturising and nourishing your skin. Add three to five drops of essential oil to 10ml of massage base oil and apply a fine layer over the skin. One drop of essential oil in 10mls of massage base oil is appropriate for children 5 years and younger.

AROMA MEDI CREAM

Add two drops in total of one or two essential oils to a neutral base cream, eg Sorbolene. Mix thoroughly and apply a small amount over the area of discomfort. You may choose to make up a small amount of this cream into a 15ml jar. Make sure the jar is tightly sealed and store in a cool place; a refrigerator in hot climates.

AROMATIC OILING

This method is very similar to Aromatic Massage, the only difference is there is absolutely no pressure applied to the skin. Your essential oil blend is gently smoothed over and left to be absorbed by the body.

This is an ideal treatment when the body feels tender, inflamed or injured, eg over varicose veins, as long as the skin is unbroken.

AROMATIC SWAB

Disperse 2-3 drops of your chosen essential oils onto a cotton bud and apply neat to the affected area. Ideal for mouth ulcers, burns, cold sores, bites, stings and small infections such as splinters and pimples.

AROMATIC WASH

Fill 100ml amber glass aromatherapy blending bottle with distilled or purified water and dispense 2 drops in total of your chosen essential oils into the water. Tighten the lid and shake the bottle well. Ideally leave in the refrigerator for 24 hours before use.

Take several cottonwool balls and fill them with the aromatic water. Gently squeeze them over the cut or grazed skin to cleanse the area before drying and covering with Aromatic Gauze and a bandaid.

COMPRESS

A medi-compress is used to treat specific areas of the body. Add 3-6 drops of a chosen oil to a bowl of water, agitate the water to disperse the oil molecules. Holding the cloth taut, place and lift the cloth from the water. Apply to the area of the body requiring attention, e.g. over forehead to relieve headache, over liver for hang over, or over abdomen to relieve menstrual cramps.

For a skin care compress, add 3 - 6 drops of a chosen oil to tepid or warm water. Agitate the water, then submerge a cloth, squeezing out excess water. Press saturated cloth to the skin to give a soaking action, eg for eczema, acne or swollen joints.

DIRECT INHALATION *(For immediate relief)*:
  (a) Dispense 2 to 3 drops of your chosen oil/s onto a tissue or handkerchief.
  (b) Remove the lid of your essential oil bottle and inhale directly while bottle is approximately two centimetres away from nostrils.

FOOTBATH

To treat yourself to an aromatic footbath half fill a large stainless steel or glass bowl with warm water. Add 5mls of essential oil and test the temperature of the water before immersing your bare feet. Make yourself comfortable and soak for 10 minutes. Dry your feet thoroughly and finish the footbath by applying an aromatic blend to your feet and lower legs.

FRICTION MASSAGE

To create warmth and assist rapid penetration of the oils, dispense 2 drops of your chosen essential oil into the palm of your hand, neat. Rapidly move the hand with the oil across the affected area. This application is particularly beneficial to maximise the penetration of the oils. It specifically relates to essential oil references throughout the book, ie clary sage during menstruation.

GAUZE BANDAID

You will need a small piece of sterile gauze cut into approximately one inch square. Disperse 1 drop of an essential oil into the centre of the gauze. Allow it to soak in for approximately one minute before applying it over the site. Hold in place with surgical tape or a bandaid that will allow the skin to breath.

HAND AND BODY RENEW TREATMENT

Treatment for hands or body. Begin by wetting hands or body, then take a small amount of renew handscrub (available from In Essence, health food stores, chemists and speciality stores), add other chosen essential oils to make the treatment more personalised, drip a small amount of water onto the dry plant cellulose to moisten it into a paste and them massage over specific areas. Rinse and then towel dry.

This treatment can also be taken in the bath or shower as a regular exfoliant, leaving the skin soft and smooth.

Hot Oil Mask

Warm 5mls of massage base oil in your vaporiser and add I drop of your chosen essential oil. Protect the entire area with a suitable eye cream. Using your natural bristle brush, test the temperature of the oil on the inside of your wrist *(should be at body temperature)*. Apply your warm aromatic blend to the face and throat area (do not include the eye socket) remembering to apply the brushstrokes in an upward sweeping motion. Leave for 10-15 minutes.

To remove: Blot the skin of remaining oil with a tissue followed by a warm flannel or towel.

Medi Spritz/Aromatic Mist

Use a 100ml spritz bottle (the bottles that have a top that squirts liquid in a mist like form), fill with water and add 2 drops of essential oil. Shake well and spray on the affected area.

Mouth Wash *(adults only)*

Add I drop of essential oil to one full glass of water and mix well with a stainless steel or silver spoon. Use as a mouth wash or gargle. Especially useful for mouth ulcers, gingivitis, prevention of tooth decay, sore throats or tonsillitis. Do not swallow.

Sitz Baths

Take a large stainless steel bowl and fill with warm water, dispense 3 drops of essential oil onto the water's surface. Agitate the water well and sit in the bowl, soaking for 10 minutes. Perfect for treating the genital area, eg cystitis, thrush or vaginitis.

STEAM INHALATION

To alleviate symptoms occurring in the head or chest area. Also beneficial for shifting from one emotional state to another. Prepare a towel, your oils and a bowl of near boiling water. Add 2 – 3 drops in total of the most appropriate essential oils and place your head over the bowl. Place a towel over the head to create a canopy to trap the healing vapours. Position your face approximately 30cm from the surface of the water and breath deeply, keeping your eyes closed.

VAPORISATION/ENVIRONMENTAL FRAGRANCING

In any work or leisure environment, vaporisation can create a stimulating, concentrating, relaxing or refreshing effect as required. It is a powerful way to personalise your environment and positively affect the way you think and feel within 4 seconds. Add 8 drops in total of essential oil to the water in the top of your vaporiser. Light the candle in the base of the unit. As the water warms inhale the aromatic vapours that will fill the air. Four drops of essential oil in the vaporiser is appropriate for children 5 years and under.

WARM OIL HAIR TREATMENT

See Hot Oil Mask technique and apply the aromatic oil blend (once you have tested the temperature of the oil on the inside of your wrist) to the root of the hair with a natural bristle pastry brush. Part the hair in sections and apply to the root of the hair and scalp until the scalp is covered. Leave treatment on overnight or for a minimum of one hour. Apply shampoo to the hair before washing with water (to emulsify the oils) and rinse thoroughly.

CHAPTER THREE

THE A-Z OF AILMENTS

3

The A-Z of Ailments

HUMANS ARE CERTAINLY ONE OF LIFE'S GREAT MASTERPIECES. Intricately designed, each one of us has our own individual behaviours and temperaments, and while our physical bodies may be intrinsically alike there are subtle differences that make each of us unique. For this reason self-healing is extremely personal and valuable.

Today, society has come to rely on medical science to treat many ailments and conditions. Unfortunately, while medical science offers us much in terms of health and wellbeing, we certainly know that we can't rely on it to cure all our ailments and woes. Instead, more people are developing a greater understanding of their own individual needs, either taking it upon themselves to self-treat minor ailments and conditions, or using a myriad of preventative methods to ensure optimum good health reigns supreme first and foremost.

Aromatherapy is a wonderful preventative therapy and it also assists the body to heal itself when it is in less than peak condition. This is especially true when treating minor ailments and conditions. Essential oils, the working tools of aromatherapy, work with the body to ensure optimum health and wellbeing. A powerful resource in any situation as you will see.

After each ailment listed below, we've included a list of recommended essential oils. We'll leave it to your discretion to decide which oils to use. While essential oils may have specific properties, not all oils will suit you. If you don't like a particular oil, don't use it. If it has a particular quality you like then you're sure to find this quality in another more pleasing oil. It is a simple procedure that will open you up to your own aromatic preferences. If you desire the qualities of an oil that you have an aromatic aversion to, simply add half a drop. Be open to your own essential oil experiences.

Remember, essential oils are highly potent. Only a few drops are recommended at any one time, and it's always important to take note of toxicity levels and certain conditions, e.g. pregnancy, before using essential oils. Using your intuition and the prescribed guidelines is the safest method to use when choosing essential oils.

Note: Recommended Methods of Use are fully explained in Chapter Two.

Acne

Acne is usually associated with adolescents although it can persist well into the 20s. It's due to the overactivity of the skin's sebaceous glands and subsequent bacterial infection. The skin produces too much of the oily substance sebum which then collects dirt from the environment and provides a delightful breeding ground for bacteria. From here, blackheads form and congested hair follicles become infected causing pimples. These pimples then seep and infect the surrounding tissues.

Plenty of water and a well balanced diet with an abundance of fresh fruits and vegetables *(avoid oily and fatty foods)* is highly recommended. So too is medical assistance and counselling if the condition has been present for a long time and is causing emotional distress.

Recommended oils: Lavender, Bergamot, Geranium, Palmarosa, Sage, German Chamomile, Juniper, Petitgrain, Rosewood and Patchouli.

Recommended methods of use: Facial Compress every morning and evening to cleanse and soak skin and Hot Oil Mask once a week. Add 1 drop of essential oil to daily moisturiser. Avoid contact with eye area.

Allergy

The word allergy is used to describe an unpleasant reaction to alien proteins that the body comes into contact with. For example, pollens released from some plants and shrubs in spring can contribute to an outbreak of hay fever. *(See hay fever for specific recommendations.)*

The body's natural defence mechanisms are triggered when it detects proteins it doesn't recognise as being part of or beneficial to its structure. This occurs naturally but when we have an allergic response to something our body is taking this process to the utmost extreme.

Basic lifestyle changes are recommended when treating allergies to help boost the immune system, and if you have an allergic reaction to dust mites, make sure you wash your bedding regularly and keep dust to a minimum around the house. It's also important to take special care of yourself——time-out just for you——as stress often exacerbates most allergies, and sometimes causes them.

Recommended oils: Bergamot, Neroli, Sandalwood, German Chamomile, Roman Chamomile, Lavender and Patchouli.

Recommended methods of use: A daily morning Aromatic Massage over the entire body paying particular attention to areas of discomfort. You can make a special blend and use it for three weeks before changing the oil combination. An evening Aromatic Bath can calm and soothe the mind and emotions. Choose a variety of combinations for your bath. This will keep your body guessing, interrupting its routine response patterns.

ALOPECIA

Alopecia is simply a fancy word for baldness. It is more commonly associated with men and is predetermined by our genetic make-up. The way we handle stress, shock, trauma, illness or change can also influence how much hair we lose. Change of season can promote hair loss as well.

Today, cosmetic surgery can help many men restore a healthy head of hair. For those who aren't interested in surgery, essential oils may offer a pleasant solution. Although essential oils won't work miracles, restoring a perfect head of hair overnight, they can effectively stimulate atrophied hair follicles into producing hair growth, and are especially beneficial for those who may have hair loss from chemotherapy.

Recommended oils: Rosemary, Neroli, Lavender, Basil, Sandalwood, Juniper, Lemon, Ylang Ylang, Geranium and Cedarwood.

Recommended methods of use: Apply a Warm Oil Hair Treatment to the scalp once a week, ideally rubbing a small amount of the oils used in this treatment into the scalp every third day for a three week period. Use your vaporiser to calm and nurture yourself at home and work. Massage your scalp daily with a massage base oil (sweet almond or jojoba) to stimulate blood supply to the area.

Anorexia Nervosa

Anorexia nervosa is a complex eating disorder commonly associated with adolescent girls who won't eat and display an aversion to food. Weight loss occurs at a rapid rate and some become so ill they require hospitalisation. Social pressures and fashions that equate slimness with beauty are often the underlying causes. Also, wishing to attain an idealised vision of perfection.

Professional help is certainly required and a concerted effort to reduce all pressures is also recommended. A happy home atmosphere and loving support from friends and family will also help. Essential oils will assist stimulate appetite, and bring harmony to extreme moods.

Recommended oils: Marjoram, Thyme, Neroli, Rose, Roman Chamomile, Ginger, Black Pepper, Lavender, Fennel and Cardamon.

Recommended methods of use: Aromatic Dressing—nurturing self by means of tactile stimulation will keep you connected to your body. Aromatic Baths and Environmental Fragrancing to address emotional needs.

ANXIETY

Feeling anxious can be a perfectly normal response to a challenging situation, eg an examination or job interview. It occurs when we are feeling unsafe and as such can be quite useful. For example, if we are feeling anxious before an exam we may be motivated to study harder so we are more prepared.

However, anxiety does become a greater challenge when it stops us from moving forward in life, is prolonged or has no obvious cause. Anxiety can be triggered by job loss, relationship breakdown, serious illness, accident or death of someone close, or simply by being stuck in a traffic jam. It's the interpretation we make from what's actually happening and the emotive meaning we give to circumstances that produces the response.

Meditation, relaxation, a well balanced diet, exercise and proper sleep can help to relieve mild anxiety. It's important to relieve feelings of uneasiness and tension and provide a relaxed, nurturing and comforting state of being. Those people who are experiencing long term anxiety or anxiety disorders should seek professional help.

Recommended oils: Bergamot, Cedarwood, Cypress, Lemongrass, Marjoram, Neroli, Orange, Patchouli and Sandalwood.

Recommended methods of use: Take just two minutes each morning to Aromatically Dress your body——you too are worthy of the time you so graciously give others. Breathe in the healing vapours as you nourish your body and soothe your emotions. A morning and/or evening Aromatic Bath can also work wonders.

ARTHRITIS

Osteoarthritis is the inflammation of a joint, resulting from the normal wear and tear of ageing. It can also appear after injury or intense emotional stress. It's quite painful and restricts movement.

Rheumatoid arthritis is a systemic inflammatory disorder that progresses throughout the body. It is defined as an actual disease caused by an accumulation of waste matter in the body tissues. It results in painful, swollen joints which usually begin to appear in the fingers. Movement is restricted and there may be long periods of inactivity.

Reduce animal protein in diet and drink more water and fresh vegetable juices. Avoid stimulants such as alcohol, coffee, smoking and chocolate, and try to increase physical activity.

Recommended oils: Pine, Cypress, Lavender, Frankincense and Juniper for osteoarthritis. Black Pepper, Cinnamon, German Chamomile, Eucalyptus, Ginger, Juniper, Lavender, Lemon, Rosemary and Thyme for rheumatoid arthritis.

Recommended methods of use: Warm Compresses help to relieve the pain associated with arthritis. So too do Aromatic Massages and Baths. An Aromatic Oiling over joints and surrounding tissue daily can bring tremendous relief.

ASTHMA

Asthma causes difficulty in breathing due to airway obstruction. A person who suffers from asthma is experiencing muscle spasms in their bronchial tubes. These spasms make it more difficult for air to make its way out of the lungs. This results in wheezing attacks so commonly associated with asthma. This obstruction to the airway causes the build-up of mucous, a breeding ground for bacteria, which may result in an attack of bronchitis. Asthma attacks can be triggered by allergens, eg dust mites, animal fur or feathers. Stress and anxiety can also trigger an attack as can the common cold.

Asthma is a condition that needs to be treated medically. However, a number of essential oils can assist in opening air pathways, assisting ease of breathing.

Recommended oils: Eucalyptus, Lavender, Marjoram, Frankincense, Cypress, Geranium, Juniper, Pine and Cedarwood.

Recommended methods of use: Create a blend and rub over the chest and back for a three week period. Light your vaporiser approximately one hour before retiring and keep the doors and windows closed so you create a therapeutic environment to enhance a rejuvenating and restful sleep. Steam or Direct Inhalations prior to or during an asthma attack will relieve the symptoms.

ATHLETE'S FOOT

Athlete's foot is a fungal infection encouraged by warm, damp conditions, ie communal showers and/or sneakers. The microscopic fungi or moulds infect the outer layer of the skin, and treatment is usually a matter of trial and error. When treating athlete's foot it's important to continually clean toenails and fingernails because the minute fungus can hide itself under nails and cause repeated infections. It should be treated with essential oils that are fungicidal.

Recommended oils: Eucalyptus, Cypress, Lavender, Tea Tree and Thyme.

Recommended methods of use: Disinfect and treat your feet in an evening Footbath daily. A couple of drops of Tea Tree in the base of the shower and a few drops in the final rinse of your socks will help eradicate the bacteria. Wash sneakers regularly, too, using Tea Tree in the final rinse.

An Aromatic Medi Spritz for your shoes will also help feet recover. Use a 100ml glass spritz bottle filled with water and add 20 drops of Tea Tree and 5 drops of Thyme. Shake well and spray regularly into your sneakers.

Back Pain

There are many different reasons for back pain, and it often takes time and perseverance to find the exact cause. However, it is important to determine the source of your back pain for only then can you follow it up with proper treatment. Anything from kidney infection, degenerative spine conditions and bad posture to sporting injury, incorrect lifting or stress can cause back pain.

Treatment that can assist ease the pain and correct the problem includes aromatic massage, chiropractic, osteopathy, acupuncture, Feldenkrais and Alexander technique *(see Chapter Three for more information about each of these healing modalities)*.

Recommended oils: Ginger, Vetiver, Roman Chamomile, Clary Sage, Thyme, Rosemary, Black Pepper, Pine, Marjoram and Fennel.

Recommended methods of use: Daily Aromatic Massage over the area of discomfort and an Aromatic Bath before retiring. If discomfort doesn't ease within 48 hours, seek advice from your health practitioner.

Baldness

(see Alopecia)

Bites

The smallest insects on Earth can often be the most dangerous. The mosquito, for example, is responsible for more deaths in the world than any other animal or insect because it spreads malaria. And what can be more frustrating than lying in bed on a warm summer night and being bothered by a flighty mosquito out for its fill. While mosquito bites are usually the most common insect bites, we mustn't forget those nasty little bites that ants inflict as well as ticks and march flies. And then there's the stings—bees and wasps. Who would believe that such tiny creatures could wreak so much havoc!

Recommended oils: Lavender, Tea Tree, Patchouli, Marjoram, Eucalyptus, Peppermint and Ylang Ylang. Basil, Cedarwood and Bergamot (insect repellents).

Recommended methods of use: To keep insects away during summer burn Basil, Cedarwood or Bergamot in a vaporiser. Dispense I drop of Peppermint or Lavender neat on a cotton bud and apply directly to the mosquito bite. These and any other recommended oils can be applied to the site in an aqueous base *(see Aroma Medi Cream in Methods of Use section).*

BLISTERS

Blisters most commonly occur on the feet due to the rubbing action of shoes. They vary in size and can be very uncomfortable. If you must keep your shoes on, it's best to cover a blister with a bandaid that allows the skin to breathe. We have a tendency to cover our feet with bandaids as soon as we feel or see a blister. Wherever possible, enable the skin to breathe. Slip your shoes off whenever you can, or place a piece of gauze with a drop of essential oil on it between the blister and the bandaid. In this way you give the sore a chance to breathe. Bare feet and fresh air are the perfect remedy.

Recommended oils: Lavender, Vetiver, Tea Tree, Rosemary, Black Pepper, Marjoram, Peppermint, German Chamomile, Roman Chamomile, Eucalyptus, Palmarosa and Cypress.

Recommended methods of use: Soak feet in a Footbath each evening before retiring until the area calms. Place a Gauze Bandaid over the blister using any of the recommended oils.

BLOOD PRESSURE

Blood pressure refers to the pressure at which the blood is being pumped into the major arteries by the heart, and it varies with the heartbeat, ie is higher when the heart contracts, pumping out blood *(systole)* and lower when the heart relaxes, filling with blood from the veins *(diastole)*. Thus we have the two figures in a blood pressure reading. The average normal reading is 120 *(systole)* over 80 *(diastole)*, and from here it can vary. Blood pressure can in fact vary from moment to moment depending on the body's requirements, and this is regulated by the widening of blood vessels and arteries. However, there is one constant and this involves blood reaching the brain. No matter what the body is doing, it needs the same amount of blood each minute.

Hypertension occurs when blood pressure is high, and this can prove extremely dangerous to the heart. Low blood pressure is referred to as hypotension.

Again, lifestyle changes are usually considered for both hypertension and hypotension.

Recommended oils: For hypertension use Marjoram, Rose, Neroli, Clary Sage and Lavender. For hypotension use Rosemary, Basil, Peppermint, Lemon and Neroli.

Caution: Majoram is contra-indicated on low blood pressure. It has sedating qualities. Do not use.

Recommended methods of use: A full body Aromatic Massage once a week for three weeks and an evening Aromatic Bath daily. Vaporisation to calm the emotions and sooth the body.

BOILS

Boils often occur when the body's immune system has been lowered *(see Immune Deficiency)*. This may be due to illness or stress. Boils are not pretty to look at, resembling a mish-mash of festering pus, they are an inflamed swelling on the skin. Boils occur when bacteria invades a minute break in the skin and infect a blocked oil gland or hair follicle. Pus is produced when the body sends white blood cells to dispel invaders.

Those suffering from recurring boils need to reduce the level of toxicity in their bodies. Regular Aromatherapy Baths and Massages can assist, as well as improved dietary habits. Most boils can be treated at home but those that do not respond to simple remedies should be seen to by your health practitioner.

Recommended oils: Clary Sage, Pine, Lavender, Cedarwood, Myrrh, Lemon, Bergamot, Petitgrain and Roman Chamomile.

Recommended methods of use: Warm Compress and Aromatic Baths.

BREATHING DIFFICULTIES

Breathing problems are most commonly associated with an inflammation or build-up of mucous in the lining of the lungs. However, there may be a muscular problem around the ribs, or physical limitations associated with old age and lack of mobility. Anxiety states can also affect the way you breathe *(see Anxiety)*, and asthma certainly does *(see Asthma)*.

Symptoms include persistent cough, wheeziness, hoarseness and an inability to extend physical activity beyond minimal levels.

Rest and Steam inhalations provide immediate relief.

Keeping feet warm will also help improve breathing. Placing steam in the bedroom at night will assist sleep disturbances associated with coughing and will also help settle dust particles.

Breathing difficulties associated with croup can be relieved by aromatic stream. Closing bathroom doors and windows, putting a flannel over the shower outlet and turning on the hot tap will quickly fill the room with steam. A couple of drops of Eucalyptus, Lavender and Marjoram will quickly aid breathing.

Recommended oils: Ginger, Thyme, Rosemary, Marjoram, Basil, Peppermint, Tea Tree, Cedarwood, Fennel, Cardamon, Mandarin, Petitgrain, Cedarwood, Frankincense and Eucalyptus.

Recommended methods of use: Inhalations and regular chest rubs are ideal. A weekly full body Aromatic Massage can assist breathing.

BRONCHITIS

Bronchitis is the inflammation of the bronchial tubes resulting in a build-up of congestion. It is caused by a bacterial infection which in turn increases mucous production. It can also be initiated by smoking or air pollution, and some people know all too well of its association with the common cold when a viral infection spreads to the lungs. There are two types of bronchitis—acute and chronic. Acute bronchitis is accompanied by a fever, persistent cough and general lethargy, and lasts only a few days while chronic bronchitis is a long-term condition with no fever. Those with a permanent cough accompanied by phlegm may like to check their condition with a health practitioner.

Acute bronchitis can be quickly alleviated by rest, especially in a warm environment. Smoke and very dry air should be avoided. Chronic bronchitis should be treated by a health practitioner. Fresh foods and juices will help to stimulate the immune system, and smoking should be avoided completely.

Recommended oils: Ginger, Thyme, Sage, Rosemary, Rose, Black Pepper, Marjoram, Basil, Peppermint, Tea Tree, Lavender, Cedarwood, Fennel, Cardamon, Palmarosa, Cypress, Myrrh, Lemon, Neroli, Rosewood and Frankincense.

Recommended methods of use: Inhalations (inhaling through the mouth into the lungs) and chest and back rubs with essential oils will provide temporary relief from bronchitis. Vaporisation of essential oils will protect you further from airborne bacteria which can sometimes prolong the symptoms.

BRUISES

From a small child to a grown adult, it seems that we never become quite accustomed to moving about this planet without bumping and stumbling into things. I'm sure most of us have had to deal with the pain and discolouration of bruising at least a dozen times throughout our lives. A bruise is simply blood spilling into tissues around an injury. An icepack applied immediately to a bruise can help reduce inflammation and may also result in a less blackish blotch. Those who bruise easily should check with their health practitioner.

Recommended oils: Ginger, Black Pepper, Lemongrass, Lavender, Eucalyptus, Lemon, Tea Tree and Pine.

Recommended methods of use: Compress and Aromatic Oiling treatments with recommended oils. A Medi Spritz can assist when the injury has just occurred.

BUNIONS

A bunion is an ugly inflammation of the joint found on the big toe of the foot. If ignored it can develop into a deformity of the bones. Joints will swell as a result of wearing ill-fitting shoes, including those that are too narrow or too tight, or heels that are too high. It can be a very painful condition with the overlying skin becoming shiny and red. As a preventative it's obviously important to always wear shoes that are correctly fitted and not to wear heels that are too high. Sandals are recommended for summer and go barefoot whenever possible.

Medical treatment is necessary for the treatment of bunions.

Recommended oils: Peppermint, Rosemary, Black Pepper, Pine, Marjoram, German Chamomile, Jasmine Absolute, Petitgrain and Roman Chamomile.

Recommended methods of use: Footbath or Aromatic Massage to help relieve pain. Cool Compresses can relieve the affected area, especially from the pressure of walking in ill fitting shoes.

Burns

The pain associated even with minor burns can be extreme thus the body's extreme reaction to burns. Reflexes are immediately activated when you touch something hot, and even though you may have had your body touch a heated object for less than a second, you'll feel an immediate scorching sensation and the skin will begin to bubble. The immediate thing to do is put your burn under cold water.

Recommended oil: Lavender.

Recommended methods of use: Applying Lavender oil neat to the burn (providing the skin is unbroken) provides an effective antiseptic and may even stop the burn from blistering. Because it's an analgesic, it also reduces pain. If it is applied to a burn quickly, eventual scarring will be reduced, or may not occur at all. Remember do not apply essential oils neat or diluted over broken skin.

Immediately submerge the area of the body that is burnt into cold water. (Preferably in a basin or bowl rather than running under a tap.) Add 1 drop of Lavender per three litres of water and agitate the water surface. If it is a small burn site and if the skin is unbroken, you can use 1 drop of Lavender neat. For larger burn areas see your medical practitioner.

CARPAL TUNNEL SYNDROME

Carpal tunnel syndrome is an uncomfortable disorder that occurs in the nerve path leading from the hands to the arms. Swelling occurs in the tendons of the wrist causing the major median nerve that leads from the forearm to the hand to crush. The pain is the result of this nerve being crushed; it radiates from the forearm into the hand and down the middle fingers.

Carpal tunnel syndrome is often caused by repetitive typewriting movements, but can result from anything where your hands are being constantly used for long periods. Try to interrupt repetitive action with a different movement.

Medical assessment of this condition is important and assessment of activities that may cause harmful movements is also necessary. Some secretaries and typists intermittently squeeze a stress ball to relieve the over use of specific muscles and tendons.

Recommended oils: Ginger, Clary Sage, Rosemary, Pine, Marjoram, German Chamomile, Jasmine Absolute, Fennel and Peppermint.

Recommended methods of use: Daily Hand and Body Renew Treatment can help relieve symptoms, interspersed with variations of muscle movements.

CATARRH

Catarrh refers to the inflammation of a mucous membrane which subsequently results in the excessive production of mucus in the nose and other respiratory passages. Catarrh can be caused by an infection associated with colds and flu, or by certain irritants such as pollen or dust. Those with catarrh will feel congested.

If you suffer from catarrh, exclude dairy products and wheat from your diet for a period and note if there is any improvement. You may also be sensitive to other foods. Experiment by noticing your reactions to certain foods, especially mucous forming foods such as dairy products.

Recommended oils: Ginger, Thyme, Sandalwood, Black Pepper, Basil, Peppermint, Tea Tree, Lavender, Jasmine Absolute, Eucalyptus and Frankincense.

Recommended methods of use: Essential oils will provide relief from congestion, and also help drain excessive mucous. Daily Aromatic Massage over chest and back for 10 days and thereafter once a week. Percussion and cupping massage movements help dislodge mucous build up.

CELLULITE

Cellulite is a French word used by the beauty industry to describe the 'orange peel' affect many women, and some men, find on their thighs, hips, upper arms or buttocks. It's thought to result from water infiltrating into the body's tissues and interspersing with fat cells. Digestion problems are often a major cause of cellulite including poor assimilation of food through constipation or eating too quickly. It can also be brought on by hormonal changes occurring during puberty, pregnancy or menopause. While it is usually associated with larger women, thin women too are prone to cellulite.

To reduce the appearance of cellulite exercise regularly, drink lots of water and loofah your body daily, especially over the hip and thigh area.

Recommended oils: Lavender, Cypress and Lemon.

Recommended methods of use: Hand and Body Renew Treatment and Aromatic Massage every day for three weeks. Aromatic Dressing using different essential oil combinations keeps the body guessing and changing.

Cellulitis

Cellulitis is a medical condition resulting from an inflammation of the subcutaneous tissue due to a bacterial infection. Bacteria invades a break in the skin causing the formation of a lesion which is hot, red and tender. These lesions tend to spread and the swelling feels solid. Medical treatment is necessary for cellulitis.

Recommended oils: Tea Tree, Lavender, Cypress, Roman Chamomile and Thyme.

Recommended methods of use: Aromatic Massage, Bathing and Environmental Fragrancing to calm the nerves. Inhalation is also beneficial.

Chilblains

Chilblains are inflamed sores that appear most regularly on the hands and feet due to poor circulation. As the name suggests, chilblains occur when it is cold. The blood vessels at the surface of the skin contract when it is cold, reducing the amount of blood at the surface and also the supply of oxygen if circulation is poor. Inflamed, itchy and red skins results.

As a long term preventative circulation needs to be improved *(see Circulation below)*. Check Chapter Three for a beneficial healing modality and remember to follow the essentials for healthy living: exercise, well-balanced diet, proper sleep, etc. Keeping warm is another obvious step to take.

Recommended oils: Sandalwood, Clary Sage, Sage, Rose, Black Pepper, Tea Tree, Cedarwood, Eucalyptus, Marjoram, Lemongrass, Cypress, Lemon and Neroli.

Recommended methods of use: A warm Aromatic Bath with essential oils and an Aromatic Oiling is soothing.

CIRCULATION

Blood is responsible for transporting throughout our bodies all the necessary substances. This is true of oxygen and nutrients as well as essential oils. It is therefore essential to have a healthy circulatory system. While this system acts as a form of transportation for essential oils, it can also be enhanced by their use. *(Also see Blood Pressure.)* Exercise is essential when choosing to improve circulation. Daily exercise for 40 minutes, eg walking.

Recommended oils: Bergamot, Cedarwood, Eucalyptus, Lavender, Lemon, Lemongrass, Marjoram, Peppermint, Rosemary, Sage, Sandalwood and Tea Tree.

Recommended methods of use: Aromatic Massage, paying particular attention to the extremities (hands and feet), and Aromatic Bathing before retiring or on rising.

COLIC

Colic is caused by problems associated with the digestive system. It can be aggravated by eating overripe or underripe fruits or fermented cheeses. It may also be due to an intestinal virus or simply eating too quickly. Symptoms include acute abdominal pains.

Colic is popularly associated with children. The exact cause is not definitely known, although some attacks are thought to be associated with hunger or air or gas caught in the immature intestines. It may also be due to an allergy to cow's milk. Pain and spasm ensue as a result, causing young infants to cry to the point of exhaustion. As a preventative for adults avoid the above-mentioned foods, take meals in a relaxed manner, eat slowly and chew food well. For children, medical advice should be sought.

Recommended oils: Ginger, Clary Sage, Marjoram, Peppermint, Lavender, Fennel, Neroli and Roman Chamomile.

Recommended methods of use: Aromatic Bathing, Compress or abdominal Aromatic Massage over the area of discomfort. Remember, all abdominal massages should follow a clockwise direction.

Cold sores

(see Herpes)

Common Cold

The common cold can be defined simply as a highly contagious viral infection of the upper respiratory tract caused by any one of over 200 viruses. Coughing and sneezing spreads the infection. The symptoms vary according to the specific virus but include fever, aching muscles and joints, production of mucous, heavy or prickly eyes, sore throat and catarrh. Fatigue and depression may facilitate a cold at times. Aromatic Dressing can protect you from airborne viruses.

Symptoms can be treated with vitamin C, echinacea, chicken soup, honey and lemon drinks, garlic, ginger, chilli, etc. Taking it easy and spending a couple of days at home is also recommended. Catching a cold is often your body's way of telling you to slow down.

Recommended oils: Ginger, Vetiver, Thyme, Sage, Rosemary, Black Pepper, Pine, Marjoram, Basil, Peppermint, Tea Tree, Eucalyptus, Myrrh, Lemon, Lime, Bergamot and Rosewood.

Recommended methods of use: Hot Footbaths, chest rubs and Direct Inhalation with essential oils will assist in relieving symptoms.

Aromatic Dressing with a few of the above oils for a seven day period will help the body re-establish its defence mechanisms.

CONSTIPATION

Constipation is difficulty in defecating due to waste materials in the body becoming compacted and hard resulting in infrequency. It has a variety of causes including stress, insufficient dietary fibre, an excess in protein or poor bile flow. Prolonged constipation can lead to other conditions such as varicose veins, obesity, diverticulitis, etc. Take time to sit on the toilet and just be there with a good book for 30 minutes or so. Breathe deeply and allow your body to relax and release.

If you are constipated increase your dietary fibre intake, eat fresh fruit, brown rice and vegetables, and increase water to 2 litres a day. Exercise is vitally important and should be done regularly.

Recommended oils: Ginger, Clary Sage, Black Pepper, Fennel, Mandarin, Lemon and Lemongrass.

Recommended methods of use: Massaging the abdomen daily in a clockwise direction with essential oils will help to get things moving along. When sitting on the toilet have with you a tissue with some essential oils on it to help keep you calm and relaxed, eg Marjoram and Lavender. Breath in the aromatic vapours, taking long, slow breaths.

CRADLE CAP

Cradle cap is an unsightly crusting on the scalp due to the overactivity of the sebaceous glands under the scalp. Dried skin peels off in large lumps leaving underlying scalp raw and inflamed. If left untreated, Seborrhoeic Dermatitis may develop. Don't pick at affected area.

Recommended oils: Patchouli, Cedarwood and Lavender.

Recommended methods of use: Bathing scalp in water with a few drops of essential oils in it followed by an Aromatic Massage can assist with healing. Caution not to get the water or your massage blend near the baby's eyes. *(Also take careful note of essential oil recommendations for Infants and Children in Chapter One.)*

Prepare a 100ml bottle with a blend that uses olive oil as its base. Into the 100ml bottle add one drop only of each of the three recommended oils and apply gently each day.

CRAMPS

A cramp is a sudden involuntary contraction of a muscle or group of muscles causing acute pain. A calf cramp at night may be due to anaemia or other mineral deficiencies while stomach cramps may be due to menstrual problems *(see Menstruation)*. Writers' cramp is caused by the constant use of forearm muscles.

Cramps cause a sudden pain to occur in the muscle, immobilising the limb temporarily, resulting in stiffness and rigidity. If the cramps are associated with menstruation, you may like to consult a health professional. To prevent the onset of writers' cramp, take regular breaks when writing or working at a computer terminal. Gentle stretches are recommended to ease cramps.

Recommended oils: Ginger, Vetiver, Thyme, Clary Sage, Sage, Rosemary, Black Pepper, Pine, Marjoram, Peppermint, Lavender, Jasmine Absolute, Eucalyptus, Cypress, Mandarin and Petitgrain.

Recommended methods of use: Massage the limb or part of the body experiencing the cramp and take a relaxing Aromatic Bath. A regular Hand and Body Renew Treatment can help with circulation.

CUTS

While minor cuts may give young children the excuse to wear bandaids, they don't usually provide the most pleasant experience, especially when paper or grass is the culprit. If a cut is quite deep, applying pressure on it to stop the bleeding is recommended and once the bleeding has been controlled, apply an ice pack to the cut.

Recommended oils: Vetiver, Sage, Rosemary, Black Pepper, Pine, German Chamomile, Lavender and Eucalyptus.

Recommended methods of use: Essential oils help in healing as they are great antibacterials. Place a drop or 2 of Lavender oil on to a bandaid or bandage and place over cut. Also, try an Aromatic Wash.

CYSTITIS

Cystitis is the inflammation of the bladder due to a bacterial infection. In some cases it may be due to crystalline deposits in the urine. It is more common in women than it is in men because the urethra *(the tube that carries urine from the bladder out of the body)* is longer in men, providing the bladder with greater protection. Risk of infection is increased by sexual activity, the use of spermicides and diaphragms, pregnancy and menopause. As any woman who suffers from cystitis will verify, it's not a pleasant condition. Its symptoms include an urgency to go to the toilet only to feel a painful dribble leave the bladder.

To prevent cystitis from recurring eat foods rich in vitamin C and A, drink lots of water and avoid stimulants such as tea and coffee. Basic hygiene is also important.

Recommended oils: Sandalwood, Rose, Pine, Peppermint, German Chamomile, Lavender, Cedarwood, Ginger, Bergamot and Frankincense.

Recommended methods of use: Massage the lower abdominal area in a clockwise direction. A Lavender Aromatic Wash can be used as a hygienic wash after urinating, and a Sitz Bath to soothe local irritation.

DANDRUFF

Dandruff, tiny white specks that sprinkle the hair like icing sugar, is a common condition. It is simply scales of shedding dead skin from the scalp, and may be caused by excessive sebum or a dry scalp. It is easy to tell if you have dandruff. Just look for the tell-tale white scales on clothing and pillows.

If you do have dandruff, do not use shampoos that are too strong. Use a mild 'everyday' variety. Also, do not over dry hair with hair dryers, etc.

Recommended oils: Clary Sage, Sage, Rosemary, Patchouli, Cedarwood and Ylang Ylang.

Recommended methods of use: Apply Warm Oil Hair Treatment to scalp once a week. Also, rinse hair daily with recommended essential oils *(ie add a few drops to water)*.

DEPRESSION

Depression is a mood characterised by a low state of mind. Most people will feel unhappy when faced with a major stress in life such as the loss of a loved one, relationship breakdown, or job loss. However, depression is more than unhappiness, it's an inability to enjoy previously pleasurable activities. You may experience depression if you have unrelieved anxieties about work, your home environment or a close relationship. Symptoms include a general despondency to life and tearfulness.

Don't hesitate seeking professional help if you feel depression is severely constricting your lifestyle. In the short term, a healthy diet, exercise and avoiding alcohol can help uplift your spirits. Self-esteem and confidence boosters are the real remedies.

Recommended oils: Vetiver, Clary Sage, Rose, Basil, Tea Tree, Lime, Ylang Ylang, Rosewood and Frankincense.

Recommended methods of use: Vaporisation at home and work and regular Compresses to change your mood during the day will assist. Also, Footbaths and Inhalations. So too will Aromatic Dressing, regular Aromatic Baths and plenty of personal tender loving care. Do little things that make you feel better about yourself. Movement creates a change in perception, so you may like to go for a walk in nature.

DERMATITS

Dermatitis isn't the name of one specific condition but rather the description of a number of skin conditions that cause irritation, inflammation, redness and itching. Many forms of dermatitis are associated with allergic tendencies that are hereditary, or it may result from various animal, vegetable or chemical substances, heat or cold, dietary disturbances or an infectious disease. It shows up on the skin sometimes as an aggressive looking rash and symptoms can include itching, redness, crustiness, blisters, watery discharges, fissures or other changes in the normal condition of the skin.

It's important to determine the type of dermatitis before considering lifestyle changes. There are both wet *(weeping)* and dry *(itching)* variations.

Recommended oils: Sage, Rose, Patchouli, Peppermint, German Chamomile, Cedarwood, Eucalyptus, Palmarosa, Roman Chamomile and Rosewood.

Recommended methods of use: Aromatic Massage or Aromatic Oiling depending on the severity of symptoms and a full body massage once a week. Use a Compress on the skin if it is open, and a Hand and Body Renew Treatment on dry dermatitis once a week.

DIABETES

Diabetes is characterised by excessive urine excretion involving a serious disruption in the metabolism of carbohydrates. Its due to the insufficient production of insulin or a decline in the effectiveness of insulin. Accumulation of carbohydrates in blood stream causes fatigue, weakness and a high susceptibility to infection. It's important to follow doctor's advice accurately for continued good health and preventative measures. Dietary changes must be followed, too.

Recommended oils: Geranium, Ginger, Cypress, Lavender and Eucalyptus.

Recommended methods of use: You may be able to treat some of the symptoms of diabetes such as poor circulation, tingling and numbness effectively with an Aromatic Massage. Aromatic Bathing improves overall wellbeing.

DIARRHOEA

Diarrhoea is an unpleasant condition characterised by a watery discharge from the bowels. In the normal elimination process, much of the water contained in food waste is absorbed through the intestinal walls. However, if food passes too fast through the digestive tract then not enough water is absorbed and diarrhoea results. Food usually passes too quickly through the body due to an inflammation of the intestines. This causes the muscle of the intestinal wall to work overtime, pushing food through the stomach faster. Shock, fear, anxiety or prolonged stress may also cause diarrhoea. This is because both the endocrine and nervous systems have an influence on the functioning of the intestines.

Recommended oils: Ginger, Sandalwood, Rose, Black Pepper, Myrrh, Neroli, Roman Chamomile, Patchouli and Ylang Ylang.

Recommended methods of use: Abdominal Aromatic Massage in a gentle anti-clockwise direction can help ease symptoms. Calm yourself in an Aromatic Bath and meditate on a daily basis.

DYSMENORRHOEA

(see Menstruation)

DYSPEPSIA

(see Indigestion)

EARACHE

An earache characterised by severe pain both in the head and behind the ears may be caused by either an airborne infection or a build-up in ear canals of small amounts of fluid. Earaches commonly accompany the common cold. The pain is associated with mucous or pus building up behind the eardrum. It is always important to have earaches checked by your health practitioner.

Recommended oils: Eucalyptus, Tea Tree, Lavender and Peppermint.

Recommended methods of use: Aromatic Massage around the neck, especially the area below the ears can help ease the pain. Place a warm Compress over the ear. A hot water bottle over the ear will help ease the discomfort.

ECZEMA

Like dermatitis, eczema refers to a range of conditions with various underlying causes. It may occur due to an allergy or it could be the result of a skin irritation. It appears on the skin as an inflammation and is sometimes characterised by vesicles or scaling. Symptoms may include redness, itching, flaking, weeping skin and general distress due to the difficulty in treating this condition.

Professional treatment is required and it may take some time before relief is experienced. Strong chemical ointments may work in the short term, but are not curative and only suppress symptoms. A reduction in animal fat and dairy intake may help. Also, drink plenty of water and water rich foods to help flush your system.

Recommended oils: Sage, Rose, Patchouli, Pine, Basil, Peppermint, German Chamomile, Lavender, Myrrh and Bergamot.

Recommended methods of use: As stress is a factor of concern in most cases of eczema, using essential oils that help to reduce stress can have a positive effect. Aromatic Massage or Aromatic Oiling depending on the severity of symptoms, and a full body Aromatic Massage once a week is helpful. A Compress for weeping eczema is also beneficial.

ELBOW TENDINITIS

Elbow Tendonitis is the inflammation of the muscles and tendons around the elbow due to the repetitive use of the forearm muscles over an extended period of time. Common among tennis players so the name 'tennis elbow' is also used to describe this condition. Symptoms include pain in the arm and elbow which sometimes radiates up to the shoulder or down into the hand.

As soon as you feel pain, cease repetitive arm movements and rest arm. As a preventative, use a full arm length support bandage.

Recommended oils: Vetiver, Rosemary, Black Pepper, Pine, Jasmine Absolute, Mandarin, Petitgrain and Roman Chamomile.

Recommended methods of use: An ice Compress using essential oils can provide relief in the first 48 hours. After this use a hot Compress. Aromatic Massages are also helpful.

ENDOMETRIOSIS

Endometriosis refers to the condition where the lining of the uterus (endometrium) develops in other parts of the body, ie stray fragments from the endometrium escape and colonise the pelvic cavity. The result is lots of pain. This pain can be dull aching, spasmodic or cramping, or it may give a feeling of pressure deep in the pelvis during bowel movements, sexual intercourse and menstruation.

Reducing stress and incorporating regular exercise into your lifestyle can be helpful with some symptoms. A healthy diet and adequate levels of water are essential. Professional regular aromatherapy massage treatments are recommended.

Recommended oils: Rose, Geranium, Cypress, Roman Chamomile and Clary Sage.

Recommended methods of use: Aromatic Baths can calm the body and assist in the healing process. Abdominal Aromatic Massage is most helpful and a full body Aromatic Massage once a week is ideal. Placing a Compress over the lower abdominal area with a hot water bottle on top can help to further infuse the essential oils.

FAINTING

Fainting occurs when there isn't enough blood to the brain. This can happen after a severe emotional shock or fright when blood is directed to the abdominal area lowering the supply to the brain. Losing consciousness due to decreased blood supply to the brain is only temporary because when you fall the head is brought level with the heart restoring adequate blood supply.

Recommended oils: Vetiver, Rosemary, Black Pepper, Marjoram, Peppermint, Lemon and Rosewood.

Recommended methods of use: Placing an essential oil under the nose (Rosemary or Peppermint) either when you are feeling faint or after you have fainted assists recovery. Regular Aromatic Massage relieves stress and reduces the tendency to faint. Aromatic Dressing, changing the blend of essential oils daily, will help re-establish centredness.

FATIGUE

There are times in everyone's life when fatigue becomes a problem. This occurs when we are mentally and physically strained yet are unable to give ourselves the time to rejuvenate and relax. Our body is simply sending out a huge signal to slow down.

If after a substantial amount of rest and relaxation you are still feeling drained during the day, seek the advice of a health professional. There could be many different reasons for your tiredness including poor diet, food allergies, serious physical illness and severe emotional stress.

Recommended oils: Vetiver, Rosemary, Pine, Basil, Peppermint, Lavender, Cardamon and Petitgrain.

Recommended methods of use: Aromatic Dressings, Massages and Baths will help to uplift spirits, and use a vaporiser to enhance your mood.

FEVER

A fever is simply the body's way of fighting infection. It usually accompanies a cold or flu and occurs when you need more body heat to attack infectious cells and viruses which often do not survive in a temperature higher than the body's normal temperature. Also, because fever increases the body's processes, natural defences are strengthened. A fever is your ally and an important part of the healing process.

Recommended oils: Ginger, Sage, Rosemary, Pine, Basil, Peppermint, Eucalyptus, Lemongrass, Lemon, Lime, Ylang Ylang and Rosewood.

Recommended methods of use: Essential oils can be used to promote sweating, encouraging the fever to resolve itself. They can also be used to reduce fever. Eucalyptus is ideal for dispersing a fever. Apply, and keep re-applying, Compress to the forehead, wrists and ankles and soak in a tepid Aromatic Bath. The Compress should be applied for about 30 seconds to one minute, then submerge in Aromatic Bath before re-applying.

FLATULENCE

Like foot odour, flatulence too can be embarrassing due to the unpleasant smells associated with it. Flatulence is a condition we suffer when excessive gas in the intestinal tract is produced. This results in its being released regularly either anally or orally. The production of gas usually results from the fermentation by bacteria in the gastrointestinal tract. Certain foods can create gas, eg beans or fruit when eaten with other food groups such as carbohydrates. Inadequately chewing foods can also cause this condition. Taking in a lot of air while eating can increase this tendency, too. Flatulence may also be accompanied by pain, and can cause altered bowel movements and distension of abdomen.

If you know certain foods cause flatulence, eliminate them from your diet. Also, reduce anxiety, eat slowly, chew your food well, and don't overeat.

Recommended oils: Ginger, Rosemary, Black Pepper, Marjoram and Peppermint.

Recommended methods of use: Abdominal Aromatic Massage in a clockwise direction and an Aromatic Bath can help ease the symptoms.

FLU

Flu is the common everyday term for influenza. It's more severe than a common cold and can include intense headaches, major muscle aches, sore bones, nausea and vomiting, and a high fever. A bout of the flu is likely to have you in bed whether you like it or not. Recovery is usually longer, too. This is the common, accepted definition of flu, although some experts would disagree, saying true influenza is a more severe infection, spreading epidemically, often over a period of 10 years.

Nevertheless, today we like to use the term flu when we want to communicate to our fellow humans that what we are experiencing is more than just a cold. However, like a cold, flu can be treated most effectively at the very first sign of infection. This means stocking yourself up with vitamins, liquids, rest and fresh food.

Recommended oils: Ginger, Thyme, Sage, Rosemary, Black Pepper, Pine, Marjoram, Tea Tree, Lavender, Fennel, Lemon, Bergamot, Rosewood and Eucalyptus.

Recommended methods of use: Using a vaporiser, Steam Inhalation, Aromatic Massage, Aromatic Bathing and Compresses are most helpful to relieve the symptoms of flu.

FLUID RETENTION

As the name implies, fluid retention occurs when excess fluid is retained by the body. This causes swelling around the ankles, hands, eyes and other parts of the body. Standing for long periods of time in hot weather and long journeys may cause excess fluid to reside in the ankles. More serious causes of fluid retention include kidney or heart disease which is characterised as generalised swelling in the hands. May also occur as a post-injury condition, and pregnancy and allergic reactions are also causes. Symptoms include a soft spongy swelling around joints, making clothes and shoes feel tight.

To release excess fluid, avoid salt, refined carbohydrates, and sitting and standing for long periods. Also, increase water intake and drink between meals only. Regular exercise is also important; a 30 minute walk each day works wonders.

Recommended oils: Patchouli, Grapefruit, Juniper, Cypress, Frankincense and Fennel.

Recommended methods of use: Aromatic Dressing, Massage, Bathing and Environmental Fragrancing to calm the nerves.

FOLLICULITIS

Folliculitis is a condition of the skin where hair follicles become infected and penetrate the deeper layers of the skin, spreading rapidly. This results in skin surrounding the infected follicle becoming inflamed and tender, emitting a discharge. The infection can be transmitted by unclean instruments used for removing hair on the body. A well-trained hair-removal therapist will ensure prevention. Use of a loofah after removal of hair will stimulate blood and encourage healing. Cool essential oil compresses are also helpful.

Recommended oils: Tea Tree.

Recommended methods of use: Hand and Body Renew Treatment followed by Aromatic Massage is beneficial. Keep the skin of your body supple with Aromatic Dressing.

Foot Odour

Most people find foot odour offensive to their sense of smell, and most of us have had days when we'd prefer our feet to take a walk on their own, preferably as far away from our noses as possible. Smelly feet may simply result from wearing shoes and socks on a hot day. Obviously, feet are unable to breathe, causing them to sweat and smell. However, foot odour may also be caused by a number of fungal disorders as well as by poor dietary habits, ie too many fast foods and excessive beer consumption over a period of time.

If washing your feet and changing your socks daily doesn't provide much relief, then a change in diet may. Eat more fruits and vegetables and keep away from beer. A build up of bacteria in the shoes themselves can also perpetuate foot odour. Place cottonballs impregnated with Tea Tree into your shoes when you are not wearing them. Likewise, wash out your socks with Tea Tree in the final rinse.

Recommended oils: Sage and Tea Tree.

Recommended methods of use: Soak feet in a Footbath. Make sure you clean under your toe nails with a nail file, and use a pumice stone to file away any built up dead skin cells. Apply Aromatic Medi Spritz to shoes and feet daily.

Frigidity

Frigidity is often referred to as being unfeeling and cold when it comes to sexual relations. It has also been described as the inability for women to achieve orgasm. There could be a number of reasons for it: an insensitive partner, fear and ignorance of the female body, religious taboos or childhood trauma. Frigidity is often associated with a low self-image.

Professional help is recommended, although becoming accustomed to touching the body through self-pampering can be the first step towards overcoming frigidity.

Recommended oils: Vetiver, Clary Sage, Sandalwood, Rose, Patchouli, Black Pepper, Cardamon, Jasmine Absolute, Ylang Ylang and Rosewood.

Recommended methods of use: Aromatic Dressing: taking a few minutes each day to experience the feelings of nurturing your body tenderly. Explore what feels good, soft pressure, firm pressure, etc, and become familiar with your own sensory responses. Also, receive Aromatic Massage from others who you trust in a pre-arranged safe environment. Bathing is also recommended, and Environmental Fragrancing at home and work will warm the heart.

GALLSTONES

The gall bladder is responsible for collecting bile and squirting it out whenever the liver needs a little to help it break down fatty substances. Gallstones are like tiny pebbles in the gall bladder, forming when there is too much cholesterol or pigments in the bile. While they might start out the size of a pebble, they can grow to the size of an egg. They are not necessarily troublesome—people can have them and not even realise. However, you certainly realise when they get caught in a duct, blocking the flow of bile. When this happens you'll experience a steady, severe pain in the upper abdomen. This pain can last for as long as four hours and pain may also be felt between the shoulder blades or in the right shoulder. This may also be accompanied by nausea and vomiting. These gallstones may pass through the duct or return to the gall bladder. However, if they get stuck, more serious problems can arise.

Once you experience pain associated with gall bladders, you should visit a medical practitioner. You may be able to avoid further pain by changing your diet. In extreme cases surgery may be necessary.

Recommended oils: Lavender and Rosemary.

Recommended methods of use: Aromatic Massages and Baths can help to relieve the pain associated with gallstones. There are some wonderful cleansing programs that your Naturopath can assist you with, too.

Gingivitis

Gingivitis is the inflammation of the gums due to a bacterial infection. It's a painful condition sometimes accompanied by bleeding. You may also notice your gums softening and receding. Gingivitis is not a pleasant condition and most people will want relief from symptoms immediately.

Avoid brushing your teeth too vigorously and eating hard foods, and pay undivided attention to your mouth hygiene. Gargling helps a lot, and make sure you brush your gums as well as your teeth. This may feel tender at first, persevere to build tissue strength.

Recommended oils: Rose, Peppermint, Cypress, Lavender, Myrrh and Tea Tree.

Recommended methods of use: Use essential oils as a Mouth Wash *(add to water)*.

Gout

Gout is the accumulation of crystallised waste-products building up around the joints. This occurs because of a chemical imbalance in the body. This imbalance is unable to efficiently dispose of uric acid which subsequently forms into crystals, often lodging itself around a single joint. The most frequently affected joint is the big toe and it's a problem more common in men than women. Severe pain often accompanies gout with the joint becoming hot, red and inflamed.

Try to keep stress to a minimum and reduce intake of rich, fatty foods, and modify alcohol intake to a minimum.

Recommended oils: Juniper, Rosemary and Pine.

Recommended methods of use: Soak feet in an essential oil Footbath for pain relief. Aromatic Oiling and Aromatic Bathing are also helpful.

GRIEF

Grieving is a part of everyone's life and should be freely expressed. It's important to embrace it wholly and to allow the time to process grief as part of your personal healing. While society may sometimes skim over the process of grieving, we can embrace it into our lives as an OK and necessary emotion. There's absolutely nothing wrong with grieving over the loss of a loved one, relationship breakdown or job loss. Grieving is usually associated with loss. The only way to get through grief is to experience it and move beyond it, nurturing yourself every step of the way. Every person will process grief differently. You must allow for your own expression and not compare yourself to others.

Recommended oils: Vetiver, Sandalwood, Clary Sage, Rose, Marjoram, Peppermint, Lavender, Cedarwood, Jasmine Absolute, Cypress, Lime, Bergamot, Neroli, Roman Chamomile, Ylang Ylang and Frankincense.

Recommended methods of use: Essential oils do not dissolve grief, yet they can offer you support and tender loving care during these difficult times of your life. Aromatic Dressing, Massage and Bathing is particularly soothing and comforting, and Vaporisation is great at home and work.

HAEMORRHOIDS

Haemorrhoids are usually caused by a restriction of blood to the rectum. They can be seen around the anus and feel like hard lumpy stones under the skin, although they are actually varicose veins. They can occur during pregnancy due to pressure from the uterus, or may be the result of a diseased liver or chronic constipation.

Haemorrhoids are uncomfortable and should be treated as soon as possible so as not to cause anaemia over time. Increase water and dietary fibre intake to soften faeces and eat live yoghurt. Endeavour to lubricate them with massage base oil and ease them back inside the rectum where they belong.

Recommended oils: Sandalwood, Cedarwood, Patchouli, Cedarwood, Cypress and Bergamot.

Recommended methods of use: Sitz Bath and an Aromatic Massage over the area, gently manoeuvring the haemorrhoids back inside the anus.

HAY FEVER

Hay fever is an allergic reaction affecting the lining of the nose. Eyes and throat are often also affected. As the name suggests it is an allergic reaction to the pollen of certain grasses. But generally speaking it is also used to describe similar reactions to pollens from plants, flowers and even fungi. It commonly arises in spring when everything begins to awaken. It can be irritated by dust, chemicals and smoke.

Symptoms are similar to the common cold: watering eyes, runny nose and lots of sneezing.

Recommended oils: Lavender and Sandalwood.

Recommended methods of use: Inhalation and Aromatic Body Massage to soothe irritability.

HEADACHES

Headaches vary in intensity. At their mildest they are a persistent pain, at times throbbing, felt in particular areas of the head. Causes are numerous including flu, colds, sinusitis, stress, pre-menstrual conditions, digestive upsets and hangovers. Of course, more complex causes are associated with migraines and cluster headaches, and these should be treated medically. The pain experienced with these headaches is debilitating.

We can usually trace the cause of our headaches, but if they begin to occur without any apparent reason, often professional help should be sought.

To avoid headaches preventative measures need to be taken, eg adjusting lighting around work space, or neck exercises ensuring unimpaired blood flow to head. Stretch the head from side to side, holding your shoulders straight and using your hand to hold your head to each shoulder for a few minutes in turn.

Recommended oils: Sage, Rose, Peppermint, German Chamomile, Lavender, Eucalyptus, Basil, Tea Tree, Rosemary, Black Pepper, Juniper and Fennel.

Recommended methods of use: Use essential oils to help relieve pain but, remember, if pain persists consult a health professional. Aromatic Massage especially to scalp, neck and shoulders, Bathing and Vaporisation to relieve emotional stress. Meditation as a daily practice works wonders.

HEAD LICE

Head lice is commonly associated with childhood, and it's unlikely any child will go through their school years without experiencing these itchy little creatures roaming through their hair. The problem is they're slowly becoming resistant to chemicals that used to control them, and attempting to pick them out of the hair is simply frustrating *(as we all well know from the term nitpicking!)*.

Recommended oils: Tea Tree, Eucalyptus and Thyme.

Recommended methods of use: Make up a blend and apply this to the scalp as a Warm Oil Hair Treatment. Comb the blend through to the ends of the hair with an extremely fine hair comb. Cover the hair with a shower cap and leave in overnight. You may have to repeat this procedure over three or four days till all the eggs are removed.

HEARTBURN

Heartburn is an uncomfortable reaction to the build-up of acid in the digestive tract. Here the contents of the stomach reflux causing discomfort. It's characterised by a severe burning pain behind the sternum and recurrent gas reflux, and is the result of poor eating habits or a diet rich in acid forming foods such as sugars, fats, etc. Smoking doesn't help either.

To avoid heartburn alter diet to include more fibre and less starch, begin exercising and reduce stress. Try to avoid overeating and dairy products, too.

Recommended oils: Ginger, Sandalwood, Clary Sage, Black Pepper, Marjoram, German Chamomile, Roman Chamomile, Lavender, Cardamon, Mandarin, Bergamot and Frankincense.

Recommended methods of use: Aromatic Massage over the area of discomfort. If you have a tendency towards heartburn, blend

Peppermint and Fennel oil into a massage base oil and massage over the stomach 30 minutes prior to eating.

HERPES

Herpes Simplex I is the medical term for cold sores: those painful blisters that pop up around the mouth and nose when you have a cold or flu, or simply when your immune system is low from too much work. Some people may also find they get cold sores in either extremely hot or cold weather. Stress is often a underlying cause, too. Essential oil applied to the upcoming blister immediately, can nip the eruption in the bud, stopping it from growing in size and becoming more painful. You'll also stop it from spreading.

Herpes Simplex II refers to the same sores, this time appearing on the genitals. It is not known whether it is two viruses or simply the same one manifesting differently. Use calming oils to relieve symptoms. It is important to refrain from sexual activity when the sores become apparent.

Recommended oils: Rose, Geranium, Eucalyptus, Lavender, Tea Tree, Bergamot, and Myrrh.

Recommended methods of use: Aromatic Massage, especially to increase self-esteem and confidence. Aromatic Baths and Aromatic Swabs are also helpful to relieve the symptoms and assist the healing process.

IMMUNE DEFICIENCY

The human body is forever protecting itself from infection which arises when bacteria, viruses or fungi invade the body. These organisms are continuously entering the body and some find a permanent abode here without causing any harm. Infection arises when these organisms decide they want to reproduce, and once the body detects any threat from invading organisms, the immune system is activated. Therefore, it's essential to keep your immune system as healthy as possible.

Stress is the most common cause of immune deficiency. Your attitude to life also plays a part, ie "healthy mind, healthy body". Prolonged use of antibodies, serious illness, emotional disturbances and use of recreational drugs over a long period of time can also contribute to poor immunity. If you find yourself getting repeated infections with symptoms lingering over an extended period, you may like to concentrate on boosting your immunity, and seek support from a health care professional. Start with lots of rest and relaxation and a nourishing diet with an emphasis on fresh foods. Try to eat less meat and use essential oils for their nourishing and strengthening impact on the immune system.

Recommended oils: Sandalwood, Rose, Pine, Tea Tree, Cedarwood, Lemongrass, Ginger, Cypress, Mandarin, Petitgrain, Neroli and Rosewood.

Recommended methods of use: Aromatic Massage, Dressing, Bathing and Vaporisation are all helpful. It is important you take time out for yourself, enjoying the gifts of nature.

Impotence

Impotence happens to all men at least once in their life and although it can be terribly distressing, it doesn't suddenly mean you're less of a man. If the problem involves maintaining an erection, then it could be a physical problem, ie you're unable to get sufficient blood to the penis and keep it there. This is often a natural part of the ageing process and can be improved by adopting different positions during intercourse.

Generally, however, impotence is rarely due to a physical problem. Rather, it usually stems from an mental or emotional concern: anxiety associated with a sexual enco-unter or male sexuality in general, stress or depression. The occasional inability to get an erection needn't cause great concern, but if it's happening over an extended period and causing problems in a relationship, professional help should be sought. Excessive use of depressant drugs, including alcohol, can impair performance.

Recommended oils: Patchouli, Sandalwood, Ylang Ylang and Jasmine Absolute.

Recommended methods of use: Aromatic Dressing and Massage. A full body Aromatic Massage once a week for three weeks as a treatment procedure; Bathing and Vaporisation to address emotional feelings.

Indigestion

Indigestion occurs when the digestive system has problems breaking down foods and utilising nutrients. Symptoms include abdominal pain, constipation, diarrhoea and flatulence, and it usually stems from incorrect diet, eg too little fibre, and a combination of lack of exercise and stress.

If you find yourself getting recurring bouts of indigestion, avoid overeating excessively spicy foods, and eating too fast or late at night.

A regular fast is also beneficial for it enables the body to rest. Also, eat plenty of fibre.

Recommended oils: Marjoram, German Chamomile, Lavender, Lemongrass, Mandarin, Bergamot, Roman Chamomile and Ginger.

Recommended methods of use: Aromatic Massage over the area of discomfort. If you have a tendency towards indigestion, massage over the stomach *(the area under the rib cage)* 30 minutes prior to eating.

INSOMNIA

Anyone who has suffered from insomnia will know how frustrating and, at times, infuriating the inability to sleep can be, especially when we know we have a long day ahead of us and desperately need our rest. Physical reasons may be causing your insomnia, eg sedentary lifestyle, unhealthy diet, PMT and too many stimulants. If this is the case, reducing the intake of stimulants like alcohol, caffeine, etc, exercising more, and eating an early light evening meal and a balanced diet in general, can usually have a profound effect. Also, take on sleep inducing activities.

If insomnia stems from an emotional state, eg anxiety and stress, then seek the advice of a health practitioner. Yoga and meditation can often help, too. Baths and massages with essential oils are often of great assistance when it comes to peaceful slumbering. Avoid television, reading and working late into the night.

Recommended oils: Vetiver, Sandalwood, Marjoram, Rose, German Chamomile, Petitgrain and Ylang Ylang.

Recommended methods of use: Aromatic Bathing before retiring *(make sure you soak for at least 15 minutes)* and Vaporisation to set the sleep environment is very beneficial. You can create an aromatic environment up to one hour before you intend to go to bed.

Irritable Bowel Syndrome

Irritable Bowel Syndrome (IBS) is a condition where the mucous membranes of the colon become inflamed forming small pockets of inflamed tissue. This obviously irritates the bowel hence the name. IBS is said to be nearly as widespread as the common cold, but a lot less talked about, naturally. It occurs most commonly in young and middle-aged adults, and results from a combination of psychological stress, food sensitivities and overactive colon movement. Symptoms include abdominal pain, unusual bowel function (constipation or diarrhoea), intestinal gas, anxiety or depression. Foods known to contribute to this condition are coffee, tea and citrus fruits. If you think you may have IBS, test for food intolerances. Leading a balanced life with adequate sleep, exercise and rest will help relieve symptoms. Relaxation techniques, such as meditation and contemplation, will help you to deal with stress. Also, increase water intake and decrease coffee, tea and alcohol.

Recommended oils: Roman Chamomile, Marjoram, Peppermint and Lavender.

Recommended methods of use: Aromatic Massage over the abdominal area in a clockwise direction and Aromatic Bathing can assist symptoms. Make sure you leave time each day to take care of your personal needs.

JETLAG

Notice how well our bodies respond to routine? They crave for the stability associated with regular patterns such as eating, sleeping, exercising, working, etc. As day and night is a natural rhythm so too our bodies adapt to a rhythm. This is referred to as the "circadian rhythm". Our sleep and awake time is an obvious expression of the circadian rhythm and so too are many of our physiological responses including digestion, temperature changes and the production of hormones and enzymes. So by changing the body's usual trigger time, you put it out of sync and it takes it a little while to adjust.

Symptoms may include headaches, earaches, fatigue, lethargy, irritability, and lack of concentration.

To help your body better adjust to the changes try to arrive at your destination at night, avoid alcohol on the journey and do a few light exercises on the plane. Compress your skin, inhaling the aromatic molecules of Lavender and Ylang Ylang, with a hot flannel during the flights. Drink plenty of purified water with a splash of lemonade added to it to help hydrate the body. Also, when you arrive in a new time zone try to establish as soon as possible the same routine you had back home *(according to the hours of the new time zone, of course)*. You can prepare for this by setting your watch to the destination time prior to departure. If you arrive in the morning, stay up during the day and use stimulating oils to keep you alert until the evening. The reverse is recommended if you arrive in the evening.

Recommended oils: Ginger, Peppermint, Vetiver, Clary Sage, Rosemary, Black Pepper, Pine, Tea Tree, Lavender, Cardamon, Cypress, Lemon and Lime.

Recommended methods of use: During the flight use a Compress with Ylang Ylang and Lavender. On arrival in the morning have an Aromatic Bath with Rosemary and Petitgrain, in the evening place Lavender and Ylang Ylang in the bath. You can also place these oils in a vaporiser.

KIDNEYS

The kidneys are responsible for absorbing toxic wastes from the blood and then eliminating them from the body in urine. They also control the balance of potassium and sodium in the blood and regulate fluid levels in the body. If the kidneys fail to form any of these functions, life-threatening poisons can build-up in the body. The kidneys also play a role in regulating blood pressure and producing red blood cells. Symptoms that may signify sluggish kidneys include puffiness around the eyes, decreased urination, nausea that threatens vomiting and loss of appetite.

Recommended oils: Vetiver, Lemongrass, Cypress, Ginger, Rose, Black Pepper, Basil, Peppermint, Lavender, Cardamon, Sandalwood and Juniper.

Recommended methods of use: Aromatic Oiling and Compress over the kidney area. Inhalation for symptoms of nausea and eye Compress with cotton - wool pads soaked in 100mls of distilled water with 2 drops of Roman Chamomile added. Stand for 24 hours, then squeeze out gently and lay over the eyes to reduce puffiness. A daily Aromatic Bath is also restful and soothing.

LARYNGITIS

Laryngitis is, as the name suggests, an inflammation of the larynx. Sometimes caused by an airborne viral infection, laryngitis can accompany a common cold. However, it most commonly arises as a result of overusing the vocal chords. Too much shouting or smoking can also contribute to a bout of laryngitis, and it can be aggravated by dry cold air. Besides the obvious symptom of losing your voice, laryngitis may be accompanied by a sore throat, fever and excess mucous production. Laryngitis rarely lasts more than a few days. If symptoms persist seek medical attention. In the meantime keep warm, relax, resist the temptation to talk *(or trying to anyway)*, make sure the air you are breathing is moist, drink plenty of water and eat fresh food.

Recommended oils: Sandalwood, Clary Sage, Ginger, Black Pepper, Jasmine Absolute and Frankincense.

Recommended methods of use: Directly apply 2 drops of Sandalwood to either side of throat. Make up a massage blend in cold pressed oil and apply one hour after the Sandalwood application. An Aromatic Massage over throat area and a Mouth Wash to gargle is also helpful.

LIVER

After skin, the liver is the largest organ in our body. It is responsible for some of the most complex functions including metabolism, providing essential substances for the body, storing nutrients and detoxifying the body. It manufactures bile which is needed to break down fats and heparin which keeps the blood from clotting. The liver is also responsible for creating proteins for blood plasma and breaking down food, converting it into forms that the body can use. It also breaks down toxic substances, both from within and without the body, and prepares it all for excretion. Be gentle on your liver, cleansing it regularly with water, and try not to over-indulge the body with too much liquor.

Recommended oils: Rose, Rosemary, Vetiver, Sage, Lemongrass, Black Pepper, Basil, Peppermint, Lavender, Grapefruit, Lemon, Lime and Neroli.

Recommended methods of use: Aromatic Massage and Compress over the area provides relief from pain. Also apply Aromatic Dressing daily.

LOSS OF APPETITE

Loss of appetite usually accompanies illness or emotional stress. If it accompanies illness, drink lots of fluids and sip hot soup to keep up your strength. Light regular meals are best so is sunlight and keeping warm and rested.

If loss of appetite stems from an emotional concern, it's best to get to the heart of the matter, perhaps with the help of a professional health worker. In the meantime you can use essential oils to stimulate your appetite. Continue to engage your senses actively. A walk in nature, going barefoot, listening to the sounds of birds, and smelling the flowers.

Recommended oils: Roman Chamomile, Bergamot, Palmarosa and Fennel.

Recommended methods of use: Aromatic Bathing, Vaporisation and a chest rub daily is recommended. Aromatic Dressing is the most potent way to nurture your body and soul.

LOSS OF LIBIDO

Most sexual problems are of a psychological nature, contributing to a lack of sexual drive and a desire not to make love. These concerns can simply be minor and transient, stemming from stress or anxiety about life in general. Most people experience loss of libido at least a couple of times in their lives. If it is only a one off occurrence, don't be too hard on yourself. The best policy is honesty, reassuring yourself and your partner that it has nothing to do with you or them, but rather circumstance and choice.

If loss of libido is more of a concern either personally or within a relationship, talking to a skilled support person is highly recommended. Also, drinking less alcohol and avoiding recreational drugs can help. Alcohol depresses the central nervous system, reducing desire. Bring yourself in touch with your senses, activate your awareness to the here and now, and refrain from too much intellectual processing.

Recommended oils: Ylang Ylang, Patchouli, Neroli, Jasmine Absolute, Cardamon, Vetiver, Sandalwood and Rosewood.

Recommended methods of use: Aromatic Dressing daily and an Aromatic Massage from a loved one is beneficial. Also try an Aromatic Bath by yourself or with your partner before engaging in intimacy. Take time to be with one another. Gently speak, touch and listen, free from expectation. Just 'be' together, building trust and rapport.

LUNGS

The lungs, along with the skin, are responsible for carrying essential oils into the body. Essential oils are carried into the lungs via our breath. From here they take part in a specific process, finally finding their way to the bloodstream. Breathing is essential to life. Most of us have experienced uncomfortable moments when we've not been able to breathe properly. It seems as if life itself has started to fade. To keep lungs strong and healthy avoid smoking, massage your chest and do deep breathing exercises daily. Breathe in to a count of eight, hold for four, and breathe out for four; repeat.

Recommended oils: Eucalyptus, Pine, Ginger, Thyme, Cypress, Marjoram, Lavender, Fennel, Petitgrain, Cedarwood and Frankincense.

Recommended methods of use: Inhalation to clear head and lungs. Vaporisation to cleanse the environment and an Aromatic Massage over the chest and upper back area.

MEASLES

Measles is a contagious disease caused by the Morbilli virus. It is most common in childhood, although it may occur at any age. There is usually an outbreak of measles every two to three years, and it is highly contagious, spread through talking, coughing and sneezing. From initial exposure, it has an incubation period of 7 to 14 days. It is most infectious 48 hours prior to the appearance of the rash. Days 1 to 4 is the catarrhal stage with running nose, sensitive eyes, cough and high temperature. Spots begin to appear on day 3 and the rash spreads rapidly from behind the ears, over the face and body. The rash is raised, hot and itchy.

Anyone with measles has to isolate themselves for the first 7 days due to its highly contagious nature: stay in bed out of direct sunlight and drink lots of fluids.

Recommended oils: Eucalyptus, Lavender, Roman Chamomile, Geranium and German Chamomile.

Recommended methods of use: Apply a compress to reduce fever. An Aromatic Massage over chest and back is soothing and an Aromatic Medi Cream is also beneficial to relieve itching. Lavender is especially soothing.

MENOPAUSE

Menopause is that time in a woman's life when ovulation stops and menstruation ceases. It's long ceased to be considered a sign of madness: it's simply a change in the female reproductive system brought about by hormonal changes and age. Menopause can be seen as a positive stage in a woman's life. A time when she can come into her own and enjoy her creativity for all that it offers, ie not simply in terms of childbirth. Still, the symptoms associated with menopause can be uncomfortable.

The symptoms include hot flushes, heart palpitations, depression, headaches, irritability, night sweats, water retention, palpitations and dizziness. During this time of your life pay more attention to your health: increase water intake, eat more fresh foods, participate in regular gentle exercise and avoid coffee, tea and refined foods.

Some women choose to take Hormonal Replacement Treatment (HRT). Others work with natural therapies: Mother Nature offers a host of wonderful treatments. We recommend you read Leslie Kenton's book *Passage to Power*, so you can make highly informed choices.

Recommended oils: Geranium, Clary Sage, Ylang Ylang, German Chamomile, Fennel, Cypress and Roman Chamomile.

Recommended methods of use: Prepare a Compress to use regularly throughout the day. Have an Aromatic Bath nightly for a restful night's sleep. Aromatic Dressing daily is highly recommended, and balance your moods with Inhalations and Environmental Fragrancing.

MENSTRUATION

While menstruation is no longer thought of as some terrible malady, some of the symptoms associated with it can certainly be unpleasant.

Amenorrhoea refers to the absence of menstrual periods at an age when they are normally present. Gymnastics, intense sporting activity and obsessive dieting can all result in amenorrhoea. Other causes include severe emotional stress, ovarian cysts, drugs, extreme weight loss and long-distance air travel. A healthy diet, meditation and the avoidance of stimulants may encourage your periods to return. However, there may be a deeper issue to contend with, thus counselling is recommended.

Atopic vaginitis involves the inflammation of the genital walls and does not usually involve an infection. It occurs due to the decrease in the female hormone oestrogen. Symptoms include an itchy vagina, a discharge and irritability. A visit to the doctor for a thorough medical diagnosis is recommended if symptoms persist.

Dysmenorrhoea refers to the pain that accompanies menstrual periods. It can range from minor to severe discomfort and is caused by the contracting uterine muscles, working to move the blood. Pain can involve headaches, lower abdominal cramps and low back pain. Lots of rest and a warm hot water bottle are usually the best recommendations for pain. See a doctor if pain is intense. *(Also, see Pre-menstrual Tension.)*

Recommended oils: Basil, Clary Sage, Vetiver, Sage, Rosemary, Marjoram, Juniper, Jasmine Absolute, Fennel, Cypress and Myrrh.

Recommended methods of use: Abdominal Aromatic Massagein a clockwise direction over pelvic area and lower back. Also, a Compress applied to abdominal area provides relief from pain.

MIGRAINE

(see Headaches)

MORNING SICKNESS

(see Nausea)

MUMPS

Like measles, mumps occurs most often in childhood, although it's known to strike in adulthood, too. Immunisation has drastically reduced the number of cases, and it's rarely a huge concern if mumps is contracted. Adults need to be a little more careful as it could be more serious.

The mumps is caused by a virus and symptoms include fever, pain in the neck muscles and headache. Pain and swelling in the salivary glands causes the cheeks to puff out, thus the name. Avoid acidic drinks and spicy foods.

Recommended oils: Eucalyptus, Ginger, Lime, Roman Chamomile, Thyme and Sage.

Recommended methods of use: Aromatic Massage and Bathing is beneficial. Use a Eucalyptus Compress to disperse high fever and in turn reduce swelling.

MUSCLE SORENESS

Muscle soreness occurs when tiny tears appear in your muscles after demanding exercise. It is thought that lactic acid builds up in surrounding tissue, producing painful symptoms. It's nothing to be concerned about; and although it's uncomfortable, it's important to keep moving until such time as the soreness and stiffness clear. There are also other ways to reduce muscle soreness while increasing exercise gains. For example, hot and cold showers: two minutes of hot followed by two minutes of cold. Of course massage is always helpful, so is a spa. To avoid intense muscle soreness, warm up before working out. Warming up should be the prerequisite for any exercise. It helps you to avoid injury and encourages flexibility which helps reduce muscle soreness.

Recommended oils: Rosemary, Eucalyptus, Sage Lemongrass, Ginger, Black Pepper, Marjoram, Basil, Peppermint, Jasmine Absolute and Grapefruit.

Recommended methods of use: An Aromatic Massage will prepare the body for sporting activities and aid recovery. An Aromatic Bath will soothe sore muscles.

NAPPY RASH

Nappy rash is an uncomfortable condition that ranges from slight redness to extensive ulceration. Causes include lack of hygiene, use of strong soaps which cause irritation, teething which causes high levels of ammonia to occur in urine, too much carbohydrate in diet, creating stools with high acid content, changing nappy too infrequently or thrush. Avoiding any known causes will help clear up nappy rash. Also, leaving infant without nappy on for short periods during the day is most helpful.

Recommended oils: Lavender, German Chamomile, Rosewood and Roman Chamomile. *(Jojoba is a perfect base.)*

Recommended methods of use: Aromatic Oiling, Aromatic Wash, Medi Spritz and Medi Cream are all beneficial. Fresh air and sunlight (just a few minutes) are most helpful.

NAUSEA

Nausea can be described as a mild to severe stomach upset resulting from a variety of triggers. Causes include motion sickness, gastric flu, food poisoning, hangover, morning sickness or poor digestion. It's characterised by an irresistible need to empty stomach of contents. While vomiting usually relieves the discomfort associated with nausea, there are ways in which to fight nausea without vomiting. Focusing your mind on other parts of your body can sometimes be helpful. Resting, avoiding milk and identifying triggers helps to keep nausea in check. If you have prolonged nausea and are unable to recognise the triggers, visit your doctor.

Recommended oils: Peppermint, Ginger, Rosewood, Fennel, Rose and German Chamomile.

Recommended methods of use: Aromatic Massage over abdominal area in clockwise direction. Inhalation and a Compress over forehead and abdominal area will also provide relief. Inhale either Peppermint and Fennel, whichever you prefer, to help soothe acute nausea.

NERVES

(see Anxiety, Depression and Stress)

NIGHTMARES

One third of our life is spent sleeping, and like eating and drinking it's something that's difficult to avoid even when we try to because of nightmares. Nightmares are the most common sleep disturbance, occurring most often in childhood. They may reflect intense psychological stress or mean nothing at all. You may be able to avoid night mares by sleeping more, having quality restful time before retiring, and controlling allergies.

Recommended oils: Frankincense, Neroli, Marjoram, Rosewood, Ylang Ylang and Roman Chamomile.

Recommended methods of use: If sleep is unbroken try Direct Inhalation. Otherwise Vaporisation and Aromatic Bathing prior to bedtime is helpful. Someone reading or telling a melodic fairytale, and stroking the person's head and back, can aid a more restful sleep period.

NOSEBLEEDS

Minor injuries are the most common cause of nosebleeds. Other causes include high blood pressure. If you regularly get nosebleeds try increasing your intake of iron and vitamin C. If they continue and you are unsure of the cause, it's best to see your health practitioner.

Recommended oils: Cypress, Geranium and Lemon.

Recommended methods of use: Inhalation of your chosen essential oil through the nose is helpful. So too is a Compress applied over the nose and forehead.

OSTEOPOROSIS

Osteoporosis is a condition which leads to the thinning of the bones. This may occur with old age or as a result of hereditary factors. Lack of physical activity, low levels of certain hormones and inadequate levels of calcium intake all contribute to osteoporosis.

All bones erode a little as we age, yet if our body is fraught with fractures and weak spots then it may be we have osteoporosis. Symptoms include limb and back pain arising from a weakened bone structure.

Everyone is prone to osteoporosis although it's more common among women because they have lighter bones. Adhering to medical recommendations, following a diet high in protein and calcium, exercising lightly *(especially in water)*, cutting down on your salt intake and avoiding cigarettes can help slow bone loss.

Recommended oils: Petitgrain, Neroli, Lemon, Vetiver, Rosemary and Geranium.

Recommended methods of use: Aromatic Dressing and Aromatic Massage to increase muscle tone. Also, Aromatic Bathing daily as a tonic and to activate blood supply and restore a sense of personal wellbeing.

PALPITATIONS

Simply being aware of your heartbeat is a palpitation. This may be because you're focusing on it more intently or it could be that your heart is beating more forcibly than usual. This may occur after exercise or when you are frightened or anxious. With palpitations you are conscious of your heartbeat beating faster and louder, and sometimes heaviness in the throat accompanies this. If palpitations occur without any obvious cause or for a long period of time, see your doctor. Otherwise, simply avoid stimulants such as coffee and alcohol. Relaxation techniques and meditation are also helpful.

Recommended oils: Ylang Ylang, Rose, Marjoram, Peppermint, Lavender, Petitgrain, Neroli and Ylang Ylang.

Recommended methods of use: Aromatic Dressing daily and a regular Aromatic Massage for total relaxation. An Aromatic Bath nightly and use of a vaporiser in your working environment is also helpful.

PREGNANCY

Females have been blessed with the ultimate gift: the possibility of creating life. With this gift comes responsibility. A women needs to prepare and nurture herself so she can "bloom" with life. During pregnancy a woman undergoes physiological changes that can cause the symptoms of headaches, feeling faint, nausea and tiredness. Selected essential oils combined with responsible application can provide comfort and relief during this time.

Recommended oils: Don't use essential oils in first 16 weeks. During the second trimester we recommend using Lavender, Lemon, Mandarin, Bergamot, Neroli, Roman Chamomile, Bergamot, Petitgrain and Grapefruit.

Recommended methods of use:

• A daily full body Aromatic Massage with essential oils added to a massage base oil such as jojoba or Sweet Almond will help you to avoid stretch marks.

• Include a daily massage of Jojoba to the perineum to avoid tearing during labour.

• A full body Aromatic Massage once a week. *(Two drops of essential oil to 10mls of massage base oil.)*

• Daily Vaporisation.

• Aromatic Baths daily. *(Only add 4 drops of essential oil to bath.)*

Caution: *Avoid the following oils during pregnancy: Basil, Ginger, Lemongrass, Peppermint, Thyme, Marjoram, Rosemary, Rose, Clary Sage, Cypress, Fennel and Sage. When using citrus oils in the bath reduce the recommended dosage by half.*

PRE-MENSTRUAL TENSION

Pre-menstrual tension (PMT) is a complex recurrent condition occurring prior to menstruation and varying in severity from month to month. It's caused by an imbalance in hormonal levels leading up to menstruation and can include any number of the following symptoms: swollen hands, ankles abdomen, tender breasts, weight gain, oily skin, insomnia, headaches, irritability and mood swings. To avoid intensity of symptoms reduce tea, coffee, alcohol, sugar and salt intake; eat regular meals with foods rich in B vitamins; and partake in gentle exercise, eg walking, swimming, yoga. Evening primrose oil is also recommended. Meditation is highly recommended.

Recommended oils: Clary Sage, Geranium, German Chamomile, Jasmine Absolute, Mandarin and Neroli.

Recommended methods of use: Aromatic Dressing daily one week prior to menstruation. Friction Massage over abdominal area to alleviate abdominal cramping, and apply a hot water bottle to the area. Aromatic Massage over entire pelvic girdle.

PRESSURE SORES

Pressure sores occur on areas of the body where there is constant pressure and irritation: most commonly on buttocks, heels and elbows of bedridden patients. Sores develop due to poor blood supply to the skin, usually because of low activity levels. Particularly common in the elderly and infirm. The sores are red, irritating and itchy patches that may develop into ulcerations if left unattended.

Patient needs to be turned as often as possible to prevent the sores. Skin should be kept dry and clean and protective padding may be helpful in prevention.

Recommended oils: Lavender, Palmarosa and Patchouli.

Recommended methods of use: Apply a Compress to the area and use a Medi Spritz to bring soothing comfort, helping to heal the effected site.

PSORIASIS

Psoriasis is the over-production of skin cells characterised by circular patches of red and flaky skin. It usually appears on bony areas of the body, eg shins, elbows or scalp. Psoriasis may be hereditary and is usually aggravated by stress or trauma. Sunlight and ocean water help to ease symptoms. Also, eat foods rich in vitamin A and lecithin and reduce intake of animal protein and fats. Relaxation techniques and meditation can also help relieve symptoms, and evening primrose oil has been shown to help in some cases.

Recommended oils: Sage, Patchouli, Myrhh, Lavender, Palmarosa, Roman Chamomile, Rosewood, Bergamot and Mandarin

Recommended methods of use: An Aromatic Massage will assist in physical and emotional symptoms. If area is irritated Aromatic Oiling may be more appropriate. Try a Hand and Body Renew Treatment to remove dead surface cells, allowing for greater oil penetration. Aromatic Dressing daily.

RASHES

Rashes can be a symptom of any number of conditions including athlete's foot, eczema, dermatitis, allergy or any other skin dilemma. It's characterised by redness, itching, spots or blisters. Rashes can vary in degrees of intensity, and sometimes they can just appear without any known cause. If you get a rash that isn't directly related to any known cause, it may simply be your body's way of telling you to slow down, ie it could be a reaction to stress. It may have been caused by a release of toxins, or be an allergic reaction to a previously safe substance. If you recognise the cause, check the appropriate entry in this book.

Recommended oils: Lavender, Sage, Rose, Rosewood, Roman Chamomile, Patchouli and Peppermint.

Recommended methods of use: Aromatic Dressing. Apply Compress or Medi Spritz over affected area. Also, Medi Cream with repeated application daily. If you feel the rash has occurred because of a particular substance, leave the skin free for a few days before applying anything.

REPETITIVE STRAIN INJURY (RSI)

Repetitive Strain Injury (RSI) is an inflammatory condition which occurs most commonly in the hands, wrists and elbows. It occurs as the result of overusing certain muscle groups, eg flexor muscles of the forearm. People most at risk are computer operators. RSI is characterised as a sharp, shooting pain in the elbows and an inability to continue with repetitive action without incurring pain. Complete rest from repetitive activities is necessary. After the initial chronic stage is over, gentle exercises are recommended to strengthen effected muscles.

Recommended oils: Ginger, Thyme, Sage, Marjoram, Lavender, Juniper and Frankincense.

Recommended methods of use: Aromatic Massage gently over the effected area and Compress to relieve pain. Resting the effected area is also important.

Scars

Many of us as children love getting scars: the result of some brave scaduffle. As we get older, our enthusiasm wanes and we attempt to avoid scarring as much as possible. Still, it's not easy. Minor injuries, misfortunes or operations can leave an eternal reminder of your past. While it may be impossible to completely stop some wounds from scarring, you can certainly encourage the healing process, assisting your skin to heal more completely. Vitamin C and zinc encourages wounds to heal faster. Moisturising with vitamin E lotion will also assist healing. A healthy lifestyle is also recommended and it's important to clean your wound daily.

Recommended oils: Lavender, Patchouli, Palmarosa Sage and Neroli.

Recommended methods of use: Apply Aromatic Swab directly onto scar tissue. Aromatic Dressing daily is also beneficial.

Seasonal Affective Disorder

For many people, the close of summer and dawning of winter usually heralds the season of discontent. It's a time when many may suffer from the "winter blues". It's not an uncommon reaction to winter, although if it really hits you hard, to the extent where you can't work or cope with life, then you might be experiencing SAD. Seasonal Affective Disorder (SAD) leaves you so lethargic that the thought of getting out of bed each day weighs heavily on your mind. Symptoms may include oversleeping, overeating and loss of libido. The causes of SAD are still trying to be determined, yet it has been found that exposure to direct light, sunlight or otherwise, can be helpful. Bushwalking or any activity where you get to see the light of day can be uplifting. Also, regular sleeping habits, meditation, yoga and milk are recommended.

Recommended oils: Rose, Clary Sage, Palmarosa, Neroli, Cedarwood and Frankincense.

Recommended methods of use: Aromatic Dressing following a morning Aromatic Bath or shower to revitalise and uplift. Use a vaporiser in home and work environment.

SINUSITIS

The sinuses act much like an amphitheatre, giving resonance to the voice. They are bony cavities that lie behind, above and at each side of the nose. When the sinuses are blocked, your voice will naturally sound dull and flat. The sinuses are lined with mucous membrane, and sinusitis refers to the condition where the mucous membrane becomes inflamed. It is characterised by severe pain in the head and neck and a persistent yellowish discharge. It can accompany the common cold, ie acute sinusitis, or the condition could be chronic. Long-term sinusitis is characterised by a dull pain in the forehead and a stuffy nose. A diet rich in fresh foods with lots of fresh fruit/vegetable juices is recommended, and it's important to undertake some form of exercise to stimulate immunity. Garlic is helpful. You may have to avoid dairy products and wheat.

Recommended oils: Palmarosa, Tea Tree, Peppermint, Eucalyptus, Marjoram and Sage.

Recommended methods of use: Steam Inhalation to clear the sinuses. Use a vaporiser for ongoing relief and Direct Inhalation for immediate relief.

SKIN

Everyone has about two square metres of skin, making it the largest organ in the body. It is comprised of thousands of components including sweat glands, blood vessels, nerve endings, sensory cells, heat and cold receptors, touch receptors, hairs and muscles.

The skin is made up of two sections: the epidermis and dermis. The epidermis is the outer section and the dermis is the lower section. The epidermis has four main layers while the dermis has two. The epidermis protects us from invasion by bacteria and is waterproof. The dermis has many functions and amongst these acts as a cushion with a good supply of fat cells which prevent the skin from wearing through in areas such as those stretched over a bony prominence. As we're well aware, there are different skin types including:

• Mature and ageing skin which is naturally occurring with age. Skin is usually very dry without either sebum or moisture and shows signs of wrinkling. Complexion is dull with reduced elasticity and hydration.

Recommended oils: Vetiver, Patchouli, Clary Sage, Rose, Geranium, Fennel, Myrrh, Orange, Neroli and Rosewood.

Recommended methods of use: Apply a skin care Compress morning and night and a skin care moisturiser daily for protection and nourishment. Carry a ready made Medi Spritz in a carry bag to top up throughout the day. *(These methods of use apply to all skin conditions.)*

• Congested or oily skin is a common condition that occurs in teenagers and is characterised by a shiny look to the skin which is oily to touch. Its usual causes include hormonal fluctuations which cause overactivity of the sebaceous glands and secreting an excess of sebum which blocks the pores. If left unchecked it can develop into acne.

NB Jojoba being a fluid wax is a perfect moisturiser because it dramatically reduces the appearance of fine lines, especially with the addition of an essential oil. *(Make sure you keep essential oils away from the eye area.)*

Recommended oils: Sage, Juniper, Rosemary, Tea Tree, Geranium, Peppermint, Petitgrain, Jasmine Absolute, Lemongrass, Cypress, Grapefruit and Cedarwood.

• Dry skin does not have surface oil to protect it from the environment. It allows the development of fine lines and wrinkles. Dry skin can become sensitive in time. It is characterised by finely textured skin that may be flaky and chapped. It may be dry and coarse to touch. Dry skin is prone to broken capillaries and is usually dehydrated and feels taut after washing.

Recommended oils: Sandalwood, Rose, Marjoram, German Chamomile, Palmarosa, Mandarin, Orange and Frankincense.

• Combination skin is characterised by cheeks that are dry or normal and an oily T-zone——forehead, nose and chin, where pimples are likely to appear.

Recommended oils: Mandarin, Lemon, Ylang Ylang, Frankincense, Tea Tree and Rosewood.

Recommended methods of use: Apply an Aromatic Swab directly onto pimples.

SLEEP

We spend about a third of our lives asleep, and its recuperative effects are vital for a productive life. It's during sleep that we rest our muscles, nerves and brain so we can awake feeling rejuvenated. During periods of sleep the body repairs itself, re-energises and prepares itself for renewed activity. It's as essential to life as air, water and food. Chamomile tea, a comfortable bed, meditation, exercise, even sex, can improve sleep. Avoid watching television as it enervates the nervous system.

Recommended oils: Lavender, Marjoram, Orange, Neroli, Ylang Ylang, Rosewood, Roman Chamomile and Mandarin.

Recommended methods of use: Aromatic Bathing at the end of the day to prepare the body and mind for sleep. Also, use a vaporiser in the bedroom to set the environment for rest. Aromatic Massage in the evening also promotes a good night sleep.

SPRAINS

A sprain is a joint injury, ie the ligament that supports the joint has been damaged. As a result the joint will swell and be quite painful, preventing it from being used in its normal capacity. The best cure for a sprain is rest.

Recommended oils: Clary Sage, Juniper, Rosemary, Marjoram, Lavender, Jasmine Absolute and Grapefruit.

Recommended methods of use: Aromatic Oiling if you're unable to massage and strap the area. Compress regularly at half hour intervals, and cold Compress with water that has essential oils added to it. Aromatic Massage when initial swelling has gone down.

STOMACH

(see Indigestion or Nausea)

STRESS

Stress is a difficult condition to measure. It usually results from intense emotional, mental or physical pressure, and individual responses will vary according to tolerance levels. Everyone needs a certain amount of stress for their body to function normally, yet too much stress can lead to headaches, high blood pressure, apathy, digestive upsets, depression and respiratory conditions. Over time it may also lead to more chronic illnesses. It is important for us to use stress and not have stress use us. To combat stress it's important to identify and remove known stressors as soon as possible—people, situations, environments, ways of being... whatever they may be. Also, resist fighting stress with coffee and tobacco. Yoga, meditation and breathing practices are wonderful aides.

Recommended oils: Sandalwood, Clary Sage, Rose, Patchouli, Geranium, Marjoram, German Chamomile, Lavender, Juniper, Fennel, Bergamot and Petitgrain.

Recommended methods of use: Aromatic Bathing to complete the day and prepare for a restful sleep. Use a vaporiser to quieten the senses and Aromatic Dressing to prepare your body, mind and emotions for the day ahead. Aromatic Massage in the evening is calming, especially when it's the touch of a loved one.

STRETCH MARKS

Stretch marks are characterised by red lines appearing on the body. They become white over time, and are due to pregnancy, puberty, obesity or weight loss. They usually appear around the buttocks, thighs and stomach and everyone is prone to them. There are no absolute cures, although you can reduce the signs of stretch marks after they first appear by massage and following a healthy lifestyle, ie a well balanced diet and exercise.

Recommended oils: Sandalwood, Mandarin, Lemon, Jasmine Absolute, Neroli, Lavender and Orange.

Recommended methods of use: Aromatic Dressing daily. Exercise and body toning techniques are most effective, especially when combined with essential oils.

SUNBURN

Sunburn is caused by the sun's UV rays and is more likely to occur at the beach or when you are involved in water-related activities. Apart from direct exposure to the sun, the reflection off the water or sand can give you an increased dose of ultraviolet radiation. The best way to treat sunburn is to prevent it. Wear sunscreen with an SPF of 15+ whenever you go out into the sun and wear a hat, sunglasses and a long sleeve shirt. If you do become sun burnt, aloe vera provides the best relief. Some sun on your body for short intervals *(just a few minutes nude)* can be very therapeutic.

Recommended oils: Lavender, Rosewood, Rose and German Chamomile.

Recommended methods of use: Aromatic Oiling once initial heat has subsided. Apply Medi Spritz over the affected area. Lavender is excellent.

THRUSH

Thrush is a fungal infection effecting the mucous membrane of the vagina. The fungus responsible is Candida albicans, and the symptoms include inflammation, itchiness and a thick vaginal discharge. Avoid all foods that contain yeast (breads, vegemite, wine, etc) and refined carbohydrates. Eat natural yoghurt and iron rich foods.

Recommended oils: Tea Tree, Lavender, Eucalyptus, Palmarosa, Myrrh and Rosewood.

Recommended methods of use: Douche daily. Also, Aromatic Dressing daily and a Sitz Bath.

TINNITUS

Tinnitus is a subjective experience that involves hearing a sound, ringing or noise in the ear when no such external physical sound is present. There are many causes and they are mostly associated with something going wrong with the ear such as a build-up of wax against the ear drum. Most common cause is exposure to excessively loud sounds, eg shooting, chainsaws, rock concerts and industrial noise. It may also be caused by jaw joint damage. It's important you get a professional assessment. After this, avoidance of loud noises and participation in relaxation, meditation and stress management programs may help.

Recommended oils: Sandalwood, Clary Sage, Petitgrain, Patchouli, Fennel, Geranium, Marjoram, German Chamomile, Lavender, Juniper, Bergamot and Rose.

Recommended methods of use: Aromatic Bathing daily. Use a vaporiser to quieten the senses. Aromatic Dressing and Massage are also helpful.

Tonsillitis

The tonsils help defend against infection and are made of lymphoid tissue. Tonsillitis is the inflammation of the tonsils. It is due to an infection of the tonsils, often the streptococci bug. Repeated states of tonsillitis indicate a lowered immune system. An improvement in overall diet is often needed including vitamin supplementation.

Recommended oils: Ginger, Black Pepper, Geranium, Bergamot, German Chamomile, Tea Tree, Rosewood and Cedarwood.

Recommended methods of use: Mouth Wash three times daily for up to three days. Aromatic Dressing to build immune system and Aromatic Swab over throat. See your health care practitioner if pain persists.

Toothache

A toothache is often caused by bacteria and decay penetrating the tissue at the tooth's centre. The pain is often deep, sharp and throbbing. Other reasons for toothache include gum disease, tooth fractures or sinus infections. To avoid toothache, brush and floss daily, and visit a dentist at least once a year. It's preferable to do this at all times and not only when pain strikes. Placing a clove into the cavity of the painful tooth may help to relieve pain. You can also try swishing some warm salt water around your mouth.

Recommended oils: Ginger, Peppermint, Black Pepper and Lavender.

Recommended methods of use: Apply Aromatic Swab directly onto the area. *(Peppermint is a natural analgesic because of the natural menthol constituent.)* A Mouth Wash is also recommended.

ULCERS (MOUTH)

Mouth ulcers are hard, round lumps that show up on the tongue and inside the mouth. Causes are varied including fungal infection, allergy, poor diet, vitamin C deficiency, or inadvertently biting the tongue or the inside of the mouth. They may also be the result of lowered immunity. Vitamins and a good diet will help to prevent ulcers from occurring.

Recommended oils: Myrrh, Tea Tree, Marjoram and Roman Chamomile.

Recommended methods of use: Apply Aromatic Swab directly onto the area. Also, Mouth Wash twice daily.

URINARY TRACT INFECTIONS

Urinary Tract Infections (UTIs) refer to a variety of conditions caused by bacteria. A UTI typically develops when bacteria from the rectal area colonises with the vagina, enters the urethra and ascends into the bladder, causing infection. UTIs are rare in men because the opening of the urethra is a considerable distance from the rectal area. In approximately 80 to 95 per cent of cases, the bacteria responsible for infection is Escherichia coli (E. coli). To protect against UTIs, physicians recommend urinating after sexual intercourse, drinking a lot of fluid and never wiping from the anus towards the vagina after going to the toilet.

Recommended oils: Sandalwood, Basil, Peppermint, Lavender, Palmarosa, Cedarwood and Frankincense.

Recommended methods of use: Sitz Bath daily. Aromatic Wash all around the mucous membrane of the genital area.

Varicose Veins

Varicose veins are veins in the legs that are swollen and twisted. They appear as red or blue bulges, and can be extremely painful. They are usually a symptom of poor circulation. The main causes include prolonged standing, poor nutrition and obesity. They may also be hereditary. Yoga, putting your feet up, strengthening your legs, reducing your salt intake and watching your weight can help alleviate the pain associated with varicose veins.

> *Recommended oils:* Vetiver, Neroli, Cypress, Sandalwood, Clary Sage, Rosemary, Basil, Lemon and Bergamot.

> *Recommended methods of use:* Aromatic Oiling daily over the area. Compress to the area to reduce inflammation and swelling. Light Aromatic Massage daily, stroking upward only.

Varicose Ulcers

Varicose ulcers refer to the ulceration that occurs over the top of a varicose vein. They are traditionally very difficult to heal, and are caused by an inadequate supply of oxygen to the skin over a period of time due to an underlying varicose vein.

A varicose ulcer will begin as a discolouration of the skin which eventually progresses to a break in the skin appearing as an open wound. It is often painless until knocked, and then it becomes extremely painful.

To avoid varicose ulcers, care for the legs is important, especially if varicose veins are present. Avoid stimulants in the diet such as coffee, tea, salt, sugar, vinegar and alcohol, and dairy products.

Recommended oils: Rosemary, German Chamomile, Patchouli, Bergamot and Frankincense.

Recommended methods of use: Aromatic Oiling over unbroken skin. Also, a Compress directly on the area.

WARTS

Contrary to fairytale folklore, you don't get warts from kissing a toad. Warts are simply caused by a viral infection. Warts will disappear in time as the body develops immunity to it. To hurry its disappearance try suffocating it with duct or adhesive tape, making absolutely sure it can't breath. Leave the tape on until the warts have disappeared. You may even like to try 'imagining' them gone. Simple focus daily on your warts for five minutes, imagining they are getting smaller and smaller. A direct application of Thyme and Lemon onto a cotton bud and applied neat morning and night is most effective. Be careful not to apply this combination *(especially Thyme)* neat to the surrounding skin as it will produce a burning sensation. If this is likely to occur you can dilute the essential oil with a massage base oil, or simply wait for the sensation to pass *(15-20 minutes)*.

Recommended oils: Lemon, Thyme, Eucalyptus and Lime.

Recommended methods of use: Aromatic Swab morning and night.

CHAPTER FOUR

NATURAL THERAPIES

4

Natural Therapies

EALING THE "WHOLE" IS BECOMING INCREASINGLY POPULAR
and more people are incorporating different natural therapies
into their life. Natural healing isn't some trendy new notion; it has
been employed by many indigenous cultures for thousands of years.
Indigenous cultures have a strong connection to Mother Earth and an
admirable understanding of natural health.

The Greek physician Hippocrates, known as the father of modern
medicine, was insightful enough to realise that the elements needed to
produce and maintain health were natural, and they included hygiene,
a calm balanced mental state, proper diet, a sound work and home
environment, and physical exercise.

Today, natural therapies are recognised on the basis that they don't just observe the physical but also take into consideration the emotional and spiritual when it comes to health and healing.

The tunnel down which natural therapies is travelling is brightly lit, its route long and lush——it's a definite area of growth as we head towards the year 2000.

We've included a run down of some of the most popular natural therapies available today. In this way, you can make up your own mind when it comes to choosing the best natural therapy for your individual needs. You may then like to use this therapy in conjunction with aromatherapy for optimum wellbeing. To help you on your way we've included Aromatherapy Indications for each therapy.

Acupressure

Acupressure is based on the same philosophy as acupuncture, ie the healthy flow of chi (see below). It differs from acupuncture in that it doesn't use needles. Instead, firm fingertip pressure is applied to specific "points" of the body to relieve common ailments or conditions. It's one of the oldest forms of healing dating back as far as 300 BC. Acupressure and acupuncture both support the body's natural ability to heal itself.

Recommended for: constipation, asthma, fatigue, pain relief and headaches.

AROMATHERAPY INDICATIONS

Many acupressure therapists work with essential oils on specific acupressure points to enhance the treatment's potential. We recommend the following essential oils as a preliminary guideline to effectively work with balancing each of the meridians listed. These recommendations are suitable for both acupressure and acupuncture treatments. *(See following chart.)*

MERIDIAN	ESSENTIAL OILS
CENTRAL NERVOUS SYSTEM (Brain)	Basil, Bergamot, Cypress, Frankincense, Geranium, Juniper, Lavender, Lemongrass, Myrrh, Neroli, Palmarosa, Petitgrain, Peppermint, Rosemary, Rosewood, Sandalwood, Tea Tree
GOVERNING (SPINE/CFS)	Jasmine Absolute, Myrrh, Sage
STOMACH	Black Pepper, Basil, Cardamon, Lime, Bergamot, Tea Tree, Vetiver, German Chamomile, Clary Sage, Cypress, Eucalyptus, Fennel, Geranium, Juniper, Lavender, Lemongrass, Marjoram, Neroli, Orange, Peppermint, Rose, Rosemary, Sage, Sandalwood
SPLEEN (Pancreas)	Mandarin
HEART	Frankincense, Neroli, Petitgrain, Rose, Rosemary, Sandalwood, Ylang Ylang

MERIDIAN	ESSENTIAL OILS
SMALL INTESTINE	Basil, Cardamon, Fennel, Frankincense, Geranium, Juniper, Lavender, Marjoram, Neroli, Peppermint, Rose, Rosemary, Sandalwood, Tea Tree, Vetiver
BLADDER	Clary Sage, Cypress, Frankincense, Juniper, Lavender, Rosemary, Rosewood
KIDNEY	Fennel, Ginger, Frankincense, Juniper, Rose, Sage, Sandalwood
CIRCULATION	Jasmine Absolute, Lime, Cardamon, Ginger, Grapefruit, German Chamomile, Roman Chamomile, Lavender, Vetiver Mandarin, Marjoram, Neroli, Palmarosa, Patchouli, Petitgrain, Rose, Sandalwood, Ylang Ylang
TRIPLE WARMER (Thyroid)	Bergamot, German Chamomile, Roman Chamomile, Frankincense, Jasmine Absolute, Lavender, Lemongrass, Marjoram, Patchouli, Peppermint, Pine
GALL BLADDER	Basil, Grapefruit, Rosemary

MERIDIAN	ESSENTIAL OILS
LIVER	*Basil, German Chamomile, Clary Sage, Frankincense, Grapefruit, Lavender, Lemon, Marjoram, Orange, Pine, Rosemary*
LUNG	*Cedarwood, German Chamomile, Eucalyptus, Lavender, Lemon, Lemongrass, Lime, Marjoram, Peppermint, Pine, Rosemary, Rosewood, Thyme*
LARGE INTESTINE	*Black Pepper, Cardamon, Eucalyptus, Fennel, Mandarin, Neroli, Tea Tree*
SPLEEN	*Frankincense, Lavender, Neroli, Patchouli, Petitgrain, Rosemary, Sandalwood*
TRIPLE WARMER (Adrenals)	*Black Pepper, Neroli, Patchouli, Sage, Thyme*

Acupuncture

Practised extensively throughout the Orient and increasingly in the West, acupuncture is the one of the most popular medical systems in the world. It's an ancient system of medicine and plays an integral role in the practice of Traditional Chinese Medicine as a whole.

Maintaining the flow of "chi", an invisible energy that flows through our bodies (and through the whole universe), is the basic purpose of acupuncture. It's the free flowing nature of chi through the body that results in good health. A blockage of this vital energy can cause physical pain and distress and the beginnings of illness.

According to Chinese practice chi runs through the body along certain routes called meridians. The meridians are comprised of a number of points, and it's these points that Chinese acupuncture focuses on to bring health to the body. Fine needles are placed into acupuncture points, unblocking the meridians and freeing the energy, allowing it to flow. Treatment depends on the severity of the condition. It can start from a few treatments of between 20 minutes to an hour once or twice a week.

> *Recommended for:* anxiety, arthritis, high blood pressure, aches and pains, infertility, menstrual problems, migraines, fatigue, respiratory conditions, insomnia, allergies, digestive disturbances and urinary infections.

AROMATHERAPY INDICATIONS

Essential oils can be used neat over the acupuncture point to enhance the energetic response within the specific meridian. This is done by applying 1/2 a drop of essential oil neat over the specific points being treated, allow the essential oil to absorb for several minutes before the fine needles are used. Another way to enhance the treatment is by spraying an Aromatic Mist *(see Methods of use under Medi Spritz)* over the specific area, allowing it to absorb for several minutes before treatment. For an essential oil selection follow the recommended guidelines set out under acupressure.

—————— Alexander Technique ——————

The Alexander Technique is a method of re-educating the body and mind to overcome poor posture and movement, reducing physical and mental tension. It was created by Frederick Matthias Alexander, a Tasmanian actor born in 1869 who spent 10 years studying the movements of his body to formulate the technique. He noticed how essential neck, head and back alignment was for proper movement and functioning.

The technique helps to restore neuromuscular coordination as old, inhibiting patterns are replaced with free, more flexible movement. It's usually taught on a one-to-one basis with pupils being shown how to use muscles the way they were originally designed to work.

> *Recommended for:* stress, anxiety, depression, breathing problems, neck and back pain, circulatory disorders, digestive disturbances and muscular aches and pains.

AROMATHERAPY INDICATIONS

Environmental Fragrancing is a beautiful adjunct to this treatment. It is a positive way for you to anchor the physiological behaviours in place. Vaporise a specific blend when you participate in your Alexander session. That aromatic blend will assist you to lock in the preferred movements. Choose to use the same aromatic combination elsewhere when you wish to reinforce the movements. Some of the essential oils that support change are Cypress, Cedarwood, Eucalyptus, Rosemary, Lemon and Myrrh.

Ayurveda

Ayurveda is India's traditional medical system dating as far back as 3000 BC. Because of its history it is thought by some to be the most complete medical system in the world. Translated, Ayurveda is "science of life". Ayus is "life" and Veda is "science" or "knowledge". Ayurveda embraces a holistic form of healing. An Ayurvedic practitioner asks, "Who is my patient?" rather than, "What's wrong with my patient?"

While traditional Ayurvedic medicine takes a total approach to the human being, it doesn't necessarily focus solely on healing: prevention and maintenance of health are considered just as important.

According to Ayurveda the body and the whole universe is made up of prana. This literally translates into energy and is equivalent to the Chinese "chi". This vital energy reveals itself as earth, water, fire, air and ether. When these elements are unbalanced in the body, disease or illness can manifest. The body's energy has to be kept in balance using other energies that come in the form of breath, food, water, sunshine, exercise and sleep. Using energy in these forms to encourage optimum wellbeing doesn't mean that it's going to be utilised in the same way for everyone: they must be used in co-operation with the unique characteristics of the individual.

Ayurveda speaks specifically of three separate body types or doshas (vata, pitta, kapha), yet this doesn't mean that a person is restricted to only one body type. Although one or two may dominate, most of us are a combination of all three.

While it's important to find out your body type (by determining the type that dominates), it's even more important to determine how we react to certain foods, environments, emotions, etc. The emphasis is on the individual to get more in tune with themselves. A correct understanding of your body type will simply give you access to your genuine nature.

The vata body type depicts freedom of movement. Vata types are agile, cool, have dry skin, a thin build and are restless. They can also be easily brought back into balance.

The pitta body type characterises transformation. Pitta types have fiery emotions, such as aggression and passion, and inflammatory qualities, ie they are prone to ulcers, yet can have watery or moist attributes including perspiring skin. They possess excellent clarity and sharpness of mind.

The kapha body type characterises structure. Kapha types have solid builds, moist cool skin and strong, definitive gestures. They are sturdy, patient and calm.

Recommended for: all ailments and conditions. Ayurveda offers us a new approach to healing, putting us in touch with who we essentially are and giving us a greater understanding of our own health. This in turn helps us to make necessary lifestyle changes.

AROMATHERAPY INDICATIONS

There are specific essential oils that work well with each specific body type. The following oil combinations can be used as massage blends. Apply daily for a week as a balancing treatment, or once a week to enhance optimum health.

BALANCING BLENDS FOR EACH DOSHA

VATA

Black Pepper, Lemon, Pine
or
Clary Sage, Lemongrass, Thyme

PITTA

Bergamot, Cedarwood, Lavender
or
Lime, Neroli, Vetiver

KAPHA

Grapefruit, Petitgrain, Fennel
or
Jasmine Absolute, Mandarin, Cardamon

Chiropractic

Chiropractic was founded by Daniel David Palmer around the turn of this century. He became fascinated with the spine after he treated his office janitor for deafness by realigning bones in his spine.

Widely accepted in modern medicine, chiropractic regards the nervous system as central to good health. Pain and disease occurs when undue pressure is placed on the nervous system. To maintain health and the normal functioning of the nervous system, chiropractors concentrate on realigning displaced bones, joints, muscles and ligaments, especially around the spine. Spinal adjustments are central to the therapy: the chiropractor concentrates on improving the movement of the spinal joints, and x-rays are used to determine the client's underlying bone structure. x-rays help to diagnose a problem and determine whether chiropractic treatment will be beneficial. If a "subluxation" is found then treatment is undertaken. A "subluxation" refers to improper joint movement which in turn affects the nervous system and surrounding structures.

The chiropractor aims to bring health to the spine and musculoskeletal system using specialised manipulation of the joints which may involve a number of different movements.

> *Recommended for:* neck, back and shoulder pain, sciatica, stiff joints, sporting injuries and neuro-musculo-skeletal problems.

Aromatherapy Indications

It is important to choose a chiropractor that massages the soft tissue of the area that he or she is going to manipulate, prior to adjustment and post adjustment. You can take along your own essential oil blend and offer it for use as part of the massage experience. Just a small amount is needed to bring beneficial relief. If the therapist is concerned about the small amount of oil on the skin pre-adjustment, simply ask them to towel off any excess before they commence. Essential oils for relaxation are particularly good pre-adjustment, eg Lavender and Marjoram, and German Chamomile for its anti-inflammatory effects.

Colonic Hydrotherapy

Colonic therapy promotes the healthy function of the colon. Its aim is to balance body chemistry, eliminate waste and restore proper tissue and organ function. This is achieved through placing a tube up the rectum and flushing water through it to remove toxic waste that is believed to be caked-on the colon. It differs from an enema which uses water to clean the lower bowel, and not the colon, of built-up faeces.

The benefits of colonic hydrotherapy are often questioned. While some people report weight loss, increased energy and clearer, more vibrant skin, others have reported no such advantages. Furthermore, colonic hydrotherapy can strip the bowel of beneficial bacteria: bacteria that is necessary for the healthy functioning of the gut.

> *Recommended for:* only for special circumstances. Because of the negatives involved, practitioners avoid colonic hydrotherapy. If you were to get it done, make sure it's by a highly trained professional. It is important to follow through with the after care program that is recommended to rebalance the flora of the colon.

AROMATHERAPY INDICATIONS

To enhance this therapy use essential oils in the water. Just one drop of Tea Tree dispensed into several litres of water will contribute to overall wellbeing. Make sure you Dress Aromatically *(see Methods of Use)* for seven days after each treatment. Apply your blend over the abdominal area in a clock wise direction. This will assist your body to quickly rebalance. Ideal oils are Tea Tree, Sage, Myrrh and German Chamomile.

Feldenkrais

Israeli scientist Moshe Feldenkrais developed Feldenkrais based on the premise that improving posture can change inappropriate muscular and physiological function. It's similar to the Alexander Technique in that it concentrates on correct posture. From a deep desire to heal his own recurring knee injury, Feldenkrais went on to develop this system of healing. It can be applied in two ways.

A trained practitioner can gently manipulate the body in a one-on-one session that lasts 45-60 minutes. This encourages the body to adopt a new approach to movement. The idea is to reprogram the brain via information fed directly to the nervous system so movements are made more efficiently.

The second application is known as awareness through movement. This is taught in groups where students are shown a number of specific movements which they follow. The student is encouraged to remain focused on what the body is doing. Movements need not be exaggerated. With realisation, simply lifting the arm a few centimetres from the body can tell an individual whether they are moving their body correctly. If not, they can re-train their body to move in a way that is not going to bring tension and pain.

Like the Alexander Technique, actors, dancers and performers find Feldenkrais beneficial.

> *Recommended for:* conditions where movement has been lost, arthritis, pain, spinal problems and musculo-skeletal injuries.

Aromatherapy Indications

Once again Environmental Fragrancing is a beautiful adjunct to this treatment for it is a positive way to anchor the physiological behaviours. You may like to make up a massage blend and wear it to the session, especially if you are receiving a gentle manipulation, or vaporise a specific blend while you work through your discourse in movement. The aromatic blend will assist you to lock in the preferred movements. You may even use some essential oils on a wrist band and smell them prior to performing the preferred movement. This same aromatic combination smelt elsewhere will link you through aromatic association back to the previous experience and therefore help reinforce the new movements. Choose essential oils that you most relate to. There are several essential oils that are harmonising to the system, some of which one Frankincense, Geranium, Lavender, Neroli, Palmarosa and Petitgrain.

Herbal Medicine

Herbal medicine is the most ancient form of health care known to humankind; it involves the use of plants to bring about healing. A herbalist considers a healing herb every plant with medicinal qualities. The word 'herb' comes from the Latin for grass and although, technically, herbs are seen as plants other than shrubs or trees, many shrubs and trees are used in herbal healing.

Herbs are considered to work by assisting the body's own ability to fight disease and are considered to act biochemically, triggering neurochemical responses in the body. Taken in moderate doses for long enough, these biochemical responses are said to become automatic, even after the herbs are no longer taken. Herbs can work in the body by improving the whole immune system. They work in synergy with the body and are very gentle. The properties of herbs have a powerful ability to draw out the body's toxins.

There are minimal side effects associated with herbal healing: herbs are more easily tolerated by the body. There is also minimal drug interaction, meaning that where, for example alcohol, or certain prescriptions cannot be used in conjunction with some Western drugs because of adverse reactions or counteractions, this is not the case with herbal medicine.

Recommended for: allergies, digestive concerns, headaches, respiratory problems, sleeping disorders, menstrual problems, menopausal concerns and skin diseases.

AROMATHERAPY INDICATIONS

Essential oils are of the plant, but not the plant in its entirety. You can use essential oils to enhance any herbal therapy treatment. Aromatic Baths, Aromatic Dressing and Environmental Fragrancing are three of the preferred methods of use. Either choose essential oils that you believe will enhance the herbal therapy, or consult your therapist and ask for their recommendations. Because herbal therapy programs are setout over a longer period of time compared to an aromatherapy program *(several weeks)*, it is recommended that you use essential oils as a booster to the herbal program. An aromatic bath every second or third day, aromatic dressing once a week, and Environmental Fragrancing daily may be some of the choices you make. Two tonic oils are Cypress and Rosemary; sedating oils include Lavender and Marjoram; destressors, Jasmine Absolute and Geranium; and Healing, Rose and Roman Chamomile.

Homoeopathy

Developed in Germany by Samuel Hahnemann nearly 200 years ago, homoeopathy is now widely accepted in Europe as a viable form of medicine. In Australia, it is slowly gaining greater acceptance as more people recognise its inherent power to heal.

Homoeopathy is based on the principle of "like cures like", also known as the Law of Similars which states that a homoeopathic remedy that produces a set of symptoms in a healthy person will relieve those symptoms in a sick person.

The philosophy of homoeopathy is that symptoms are signs of the body's effort to throw off disease. Minute doses of biological substances are used to stimulate healing in the body. A professional homoeopath can formulate homoeopathic remedies which are individually tailored to the client's specific needs for maintaining health. Because homoeopathic medicines are so highly diluted, there is little danger of toxicity or side-effects. As a result, they are considered safe to use in the home and are valuable in the treatment of domestic illnesses and for treating children.

> *Recommended for:* colds and flu, allergies, catarrh, depression, stress, cold sores, travel sickness, and much else including acute, chronic, physical, emotional and inherited diseases. How effective treatment is will depend on the individual.

AROMATHERAPY INDICATIONS

There are different views about the use of aromatherapy in conjunction with homoeopathy. One view is you should never blend the two modalities, because the essential oils neutralise the homoeopathics. The other is that you can combine the two with certain essential oils. The choice is ultimately up to you––go with what you feel is best.

Our view is that you can blend the two modalities. We advocate certain guidelines. First, store both your homoeopathic preparations and essential oils in different locations (cupboards and/or rooms). Second, we recommend you avoid using the following essential oils from the 40 we recommend for use in Chapter One with any homoeopathic preparations: Peppermint, Rosemary, Eucalyptus, Tea Tree and Thyme.

───────────── Hydrotherapy ─────────────

Water has long been recognised for its healing benefits. Documented evidence suggests Hippocrates, the father of modern medicine, used water for healing purposes as far back as 460 BC. Since then many have benefited from the healing power of water whether it be by bathing in a natural spring nestled in the mountains or in the bath tub at home. Traditionally speaking hydrotherapy can be employed in many different ways including compresses, enemas and Steam Inhalations, ie any treatment that involves the use of water.

Recommended for: relaxation, pain, muscle spasm, assisting joint movement, strengthening muscles and improving circulation.

AROMATHERAPY INDICATIONS

Aromatherapy is the perfect compliment to hydrotherapy. Essential oils added into your bath, compress bowl, vaporiser, sitz bath, steam room, or foot bowl will transform the water into a treatment solution that works wonders for your health and wellbeing. Simply follow the dosage recommendations relative to your chosen method of use.

Relaxation Blend
Lavender, Bergamot, Cedarwood

Productivity and Focus
Lemon, Basil, Rosewood

Romance and Intimacy
Ylang Ylang, Orange, Patchouli

Discovery and Learning
Basil, Petitgrain, Lime

Joy and Celebration
Petitgrain, Orange, Clary Sage

Kinesiology

Kinesiology, also known as "muscle testing", is the study of muscle movement. It uses gentle muscle testing to monitor personal information about a person's wellbeing and identifies blockages in the body's natural energy flow. According to kinesiology, muscles become monitors of stress and imbalance in the body. It was developed by chiropractors in the 1960s but unlike the chiropractor a kinesiologist isn't trained to manipulate the body. A kinesiologist instead uses massage points, diet, nutrition and emotional healing to remedy diagnosed problems.

Kinesiology finds energy blockages in the body, it then concentrates on increasing energy so the body can heal itself.

Recommended for: allergies, stress, emotional disorders, bronchitis, breathing difficulties, PMS and psoriasis.

AROMATHERAPY INDICATIONS

Essential oils can be used by kinesiologists when muscle testing. Essential oils can be held by the recipient while the test is being performed, and the bottle is sometimes held over the umbilicus (belly button), too. Some aromatherapists use muscle testing as a means to further check the essential oil selection most appropriate for you. Essential oils can also be used to balance energy: this relates to the energy meridians that flow through our bodies. See acupressure for essential oil recommendations.

Massage

The question today isn't necessarily, "Should I get a massage?" but rather, "What massage should I get?" Many different massage techniques are practised including acupressure, Indian head, neck and shoulder massage, reflexology and shiatsu. *(See appropriate entries for more information.)*

There's also remedial massage which concentrates on soft body tissue, the muscles and ligaments to stimulate the circulation of blood and the functioning of the nervous system.

AROMATHERAPY INDICATIONS

Massage is the most potent way of using aromatherapy. It is the method of use that permits the essential oils to be most responsive over the longest period of time. Choosing essential oils for your massage treatment is very simple. Make your selection according to the response that you most desire, either physically, mentally, emotionally or spiritually. It is important that you like the aromatic blend for it to do you any good. If your senses repel the aroma you body will reject the healing benefits available. It doesn't have to be your favourite perfume, it just has to be acceptable to your senses.

Revive Blend
Grapefruit, Ginger, Ylang Ylang

Stress Buster Blend
Cedarwood, Neroli, Lavender

Rejuvenation Blend
Frankincense, Neroli, Lavender

Sensual Aphrodisiac Blend
Clary Sage, Patchouli, Orange, Ylang Ylang

NB Add 1 drop of oil to every 2mls of massage base oil.

Meditation

When practiced on a regular basis, meditation eases the mind and body from the stresses of everyday life. It is a form of discipline devised by sages in the East thousands of years ago to silence the 'wild roars' of the human mind.

Much of the stress we experience is associated with a confused mind. Each day we present it with at least 60,000 thoughts to contend with, and even when we sleep our mind is still active. Like everything, our mind needs rest and this can be done through meditation.

At first you may find your mind wandering when you sit down to meditate. This is only natural. After a time you will find yourself experiencing brief moments where you are fully focused on who you are with absolutely no other concerns occupying your mind.

Meditation brings you closer to yourself, giving you a better understanding of what you are meant to be doing, freeing you from frustration and confusion.

A study of Egyptian papyrus and hieroglyphics reveal that the human race has in one way or another employed the techniques of meditation and cured a host of ailments.

There are many meditations to choose from including primordial sound meditation, transcendental meditation, mantra meditation, synchronicity high-tech meditation and zazen.

Recommended for: everything. Make it a part of your everyday life.

AROMATHERAPY INDICATIONS

Environmental Fragrancing is the preferred method of use for enhancing your meditation practice. Choose from your wardrobe of essential oils to focus, centre or quieten. People who choose to meditate in the bath will receive the benefits from hydrotherapy as well. Simply follow the Methods of Use *(Chapter Two)* for drops and dosage requirements so you truly receive the healing benefits.

Early Morning Meditation Blend
Lemon, Black Pepper, Petitgrain

Evening Blend
Thyme, Ginger, Palmarosa, Frankincense, Juniper

Meditation and Contemplation Blend
Rose, Lavender, Frankincense, Sandalwood, Myrrh

Naturopathy

Naturopathy acknowledges, as the name suggests, that nature is the true and only healer—practitioners merely create the optimum conditions for this to occur.

Developed in Europe in the late 18th century, naturopathy deals with internal health problems, metabolic disorders and imbalances through treatment of the whole person. Naturopathy addresses the underlying cause of illness, primarily unfavourable habits or lifestyles. It deals with restoring health rather than combating disease. In naturopathy, symptoms are viewed as signs that the body is trying to heal itself.

The aim is to induce health by making the individual more resilient, improving the strength of the immune system. Naturopaths are viewed as teachers rather than doctors, working with patients and educating them about good health practices. Treatment may involve dietary changes, herbal medicines, homoeopathy, bodywork or nutritional supplementation. It is gentle and non-intrusive.

Some naturopaths will use iridology. Iridology means "a study of the eyes". It is a science, that through the eyes can reveal the health condition of the body. The iris works as a display unit of everything that takes place in our bodies. Its various colours, tissues, fibre structure and patterns all correspond to specific organs and tissues in the body and an iridologist can tell through the changes in patterns and colours the state of health of each organ in a person. Iridology cannot tell the name of a disease, but it does show inflammation, toxicity, catarrh deposits, blood supply, nerve condition, lesions or irritation. Often the cause of an ailment is found in a different location to the site of the symptom. Early indications of imminent conditions can be apparent so that appropriate treatment can be taken to prevent major ailments later in life.

Recommended for: all ailments and conditions.

AROMATHERAPY INDICATIONS

A naturopath has a wide range of natural healing modalities to choose from, and the very versatile nature of aromatherapy enables you to incorporate essential oil therapy into any facet of your treatment program. As in herbal therapy, you can use essential oils as boosters to your personal care regime: the variety of methods of use enables you to fully embrace aromatherapy, whether you are detoxifying your liver, cleansing you colon, improving you circulation, or simply endeavouring to manage your personal stress. Ask your naturopath to help you design an aromatherapy program, and be adventurous and choose for yourself, too. Aromatic Dressing from your ultimate wardrobe (*the 40 essential oils listed in Chapter One*); select three different essential oils each day for a period of three weeks. This will help change set patterns in the body's system.

Oesteopathy

Osteopathy is a bodywork therapy that combines a number of principles to help restore the structural balance of the musculo-skeletal system. It combines joint manipulation, physical therapy and postural re-education. It was developed prior to chiropractic and relies on stimulating the body's natural ability to self-heal. While the spine is central to the therapy, the diagnosis of structural problems within the musculo-skeletal system and the corresponding manipulative treatment are the most fundamental aspects of osteopathy.

An osteopath views the body as a complete unit made up of interconnective parts. When the body is healthy it is able to defend itself against injury and infection. It's also able to recover more readily from trauma. This ability to defend itself can only take place when the body is in peak condition, and according to osteopathy this can only occur when there is maximum health at a structural level. It therefore aims to correct any internal malfunctions, encouraging the body's ability to heal itself.

Osteopathy uses 'hands on' techniques such as deep tactile pressure, stretching and gentle manipulation of muscles and joints.

> *Recommended for:* back, neck and shoulder pain, headaches, other bodily aches and pains, sprains, sinus problems, sciatica and recurring strain injuries.

AROMATHERAPY INDICATIONS

An Aromatic Massage, including a brisk rub of a blend of essential oils over the spine, enhances the postural re-education that osteopathy seeks to achieve. As with any manipulative treatment, especially that which involves the soft tissue of the muscles, essential oils by their very nature assist the body's circulatory and immune response. An Aromatic Bath works wonders after any adjustments, especially to the spine. When using essential oils as part of the treatment, it is recommended to rest for up to four hours after you have received your treatment. This allows for full absorption of the essential oils and the maximum healing response. Only a small amount of your massage blend is required so that the skin doesn't become slippery prior to any adjustments. Rosemary, Lemongrass, Eucalyptus, Black Pepper, Peppermint and Juniper are some possible choices.

Polarity Therapy

Polarity Therapy is based on the premise that illnesses arise because of blockages in our energy flow. This is very much in line with Eastern thinking, ie the Chinese *chi* or Indian *prana*.

Dr Randolph Stone, a naturopath, chiropractor and osteopath, developed the therapy over a 50 year period. Polarity therapy employs a number of 'hands on' techniques for healing including massage, breathing techniques, hydrotherapy, exercise and reflexology. All techniques employed are designed to restore a healthy energy flow through the body. These techniques are combined with dietary considerations and counselling to form a holistic approach to healing.

Recommended for: allergies, respiratory problems, headaches and migraines, back pain, digestive complaints, stress and anxiety.

Aromatherapy Indications

Aromatherapy works well with a therapy that addresses our energy system. Working with the breath is essential to this particular treatment, therefore, vaporisation can be employed to calm, centre and quieten the mind during your treatment. Essential oils can be blended and used in any of the tactile hands on work. Follow up with a relaxing bath that evening before retiring. You may wish to ask you therapist which essential oil blend was used so you can recreate the aromatic combination at home and once again reconnect with the experience. Essential oils that particularly relate to respiration are Eucalyptus, Pine, Cedarwood, Peppermint and Tea Tree.

Postural Integration

Postural Integration is a slow and systematic way of loosening the deep tissue and muscles of the body. During this process, any distortion in posture is reduced and closer alignment with gravity is restored. Also, any repressed fears, needs and wants are expressed and released together with any childhood traumas. These are then integrated, helping the client towards a greater clarity of being, be it in relationships or career. A more vibrant and harmonious state of wellbeing is achieved.

This kind of bodywork is more closely associated with psychotherapy as it pays more attention to the psycho-emotional effects of physical restructuring.

Recommended for: stress, depression and anxiety.

Aromatherapy Indications

This slow deep procedure is enhanced with essential oils, especially with regard to the repair of tissue. As with any deep restructuring of muscle tissue, tiny muscle fibres tear, breaking away from the restricted form they were previously held in, ie the old patterns that produce pain or discomfort. Creating change to the area posturally while using essential oils assists in breaking physical and emotional bonds and helps to create an environment where true healing can occur. Oils that help promote change are Myrrh, Sandalwood, Frankincense, Cardamon and Rosewood.

Reflexology

Reflexology is the specific bodywork technique of stroking or applying pressure to one part of the body to affect changes in another part of the body. It can be used to relax muscles and stimulate the body's own ability to heal itself. Reflexology works on the principle that the hands and feet are a map of the complete anatomy with reflex areas corresponding to every part of the body.

Reflexologists massage specific areas to relieve tension or blockages along energy meridians which can cause pain and disease. They often target the break-up of lactic acid and calcium crystals accumulated around the 7,200 nerve endings in each foot. The nerve endings found in the feet interconnect extensively through the spinal cord and brain to all areas of the body.

In a typical session, the reflexologist holds each foot, using mainly thumbs to stroke or press the bottom, top and sides. The bottom of the foot has the more effective reflex points but working the top and sides of the foot also has benefits. The treatment will be a combination of general foot massage and pressure on specific points which may correlate to specific problem areas.

> *Recommended for:* stress, circulatory problems and release of toxins.

AROMATHERAPY INDICATIONS

Reflexologists usually use powder to move over the skin as they press the reflex points on the feet. Silk powder is the best to use; because its natural it allows the skin to breathe. One drop of essential oil *(either Sage, Tea Tree, Cypress or Juniper are ideal)* can be added to a small amount of the powder. Allow the powder to dry for a few minutes and with a gentle rubbing and crumbling action with your fingers endeavour to blend the one drop through the entire portion of powder for your treatment. If you are seeing a reflexologist you may choose to prepare your own aromatic powder at home, or pass the tip onto you therapist so they can make their own. Another way to enhance your reflexology treatment is to ask your therapist to complete the treatment with an aromatic oiling using a prescriptive aromatherapy blend. In this way, you really get to take the treatment home with you. Some choices are Sage, Juniper, Tea Tree, Cypress, Lime or Black Pepper.

Reiki

Reiki (pronounced ray-kee) was developed by Dr Mikao Usui, a Japanese Christian. It is based on ancient Tibetan knowledge Usui rediscovered in the mid 1800s. As a minister in Kyoto, Japan, Dr Usui began researching world religions for a description and understanding of Jesus' healing methods.

After learning Sanskrit, so he could read the ancient and esoteric sutras, and after years of study and meditation, Dr Usui finally uncovered the healing knowledge he sought within the symbols of the sacred Tibetan texts. Dr Usui named this rediscovered healing system from the Japanese words rei––meaning boundless and universal––and ki––the vital life force energy flowing through all living beings.

In Reiki a practitioner acts as a channel for the universal life force, which enters the body through the crown of the head, and is then experienced as a tingling sensation or a warmth, heat, chills or tremors.

A typical treatment covering all the vital areas may take an hour and a half. After a full Reiki treatment clients report a lift in vitality and mental clarity.

Recommended for: stress, fatigue, aching muscles, headaches, colds and flu, cuts, burns, stomach upsets and sprains.

AROMATHERAPY INDICATIONS

One of the simplest and effective ways to incorporate essential oil therapy into your treatment is through vaporisation. For someone giving a treatment, choose a combination of essential oils that the recipient most enjoys. If you're receiving the treatment, choose essential oils for how you want to feel. We call this choosing from the land of 'more'. I want more relaxation, abundance, self expression and confidence, love and connection, or certainty and variety. We believe that this is a 'more' empowering place to choose from, rather than less of this or that. Placing your attention on the outcome you desire when you make your essential oil selection is powerful. Then hold the intention as you embrace your treatment. Relax, breathe and receive. Choose an essential oil that is most pleasing to your senses and use that oil for the duration of the session to aromatically anchor the healing response.

Shiatsu

Shiatsu is a Japanese massage technique that literally translates into "finger pressure". It incorporates a rhythmic series of finger pressures held between three and five seconds to awaken the acupuncture meridians. It also utilises a series of stretches, thus the treatment can be stimulating as well as relaxing.

The aim is to use pressure on the right points to induce the muscles to relax, allowing the chi to flow, and promoting the body's own recuperative abilities. Shiatsu practitioners need to have a good balance of energy themselves as a strict requirement of shiatsu is that the ki or chi of the therapist is in good shape.

Rather than using a massage table, a full shiatsu is usually carried out on a futon on the floor.

Recommended for: headaches, asthma, constipation, menstrual problems, hay fever, circulatory concerns and tense muscles.

AROMATHERAPY INDICATIONS

Some Shiatsu therapists use small amounts of massage base oil to move over the surface of the skin, while others use powder or nothing at all. Refer to the reflexology section for tips on using essential oils during finger pressure therapy, ie shiatsu. To receive an Aromatic Oiling with the massage is a beneficial contribution, either on completion or during the treatment. If the oiling is received post-treatment, either you or the therapist can do it. Simply take a small amount of your blended massage oil *(see the Methods of Use section on how to make it up)* and begin at either your head or feet, working it into the skin and covering as much skin surface as you can. If you want to take your attention away from the thinking self, work from the head to the feet, and the reverse applies if you want to be mindful. Refer to the acupressure chart for the essential oils that relate to specific meridians.

—— Traditional Chinese Medicine (TMC) ——

Based on the principles of yin/yang, TMC embraces a wide range of time tested natural remedies that are thousands of years old. Diagnosis includes tongue, abdomen and pulse readings.

Medicines are used from the mineral, plant and animal kingdom. Some of the herbs used include licorice, mandarin skins, ginger, cardamon and ginseng. The herbs are usually made into special formulas. Traditionally, the herbs are simmered in a ceramic pot, but new methods of extraction have allowed them to be made into more convenient forms like granules and tablets.

Practitioners observe disharmony in the client's systems and then work to bring balance using different treatments. TMC today incorporates a wide range of treatments, including herbal medicine, acupuncture, dietary therapy and massage.

Each treatment is designed to keep a delicate balance of health, emphasising the prevention of disease rather than the masking of symptoms. TMC is a popular form of Eastern healing, practised commonly in the West.

Recommended for: all ailments and conditions.

AROMATHERAPY INDICATIONS

For centuries the Chinese have incorporated aromatic plants into their healing practices. As the plants themselves are used in medicines so too are the concentrated, volatile aromatic molecules of their corresponding essential oils. Mandarin, Ginger and Cardamon Aromatic Baths enhance the efficacy of all tradition Chinese medical treatments. Ask your therapist for their recommended method of use. Bathing may become the complementing treatment, or massage. The health enhancing qualities of pure essential oils can always be enjoyed.

Yoga

Yoga has been practised in Eastern nations for over 2,000 years and is known as the surest way to reach "the world of permanent happiness". It is derived from a set of 10 basic postures called asanas that go far beyond the famous lotus (sitting cross-legged) position. Each of the static poses focuses on a different area of the body, relaxing and stretching it to prevent injury.

Each posture acts as a counter balance to other postures to make certain balance is maintained. While some of the stretches require a degree of strength and flexibility, yoga is primarily a gentle art and is accessible to everyone. Attention is also paid to breathing exercises, meditation and relaxation.

> *Recommended for:* circulatory problems, lower back pain, stress, asthma, respiratory problems, sleeping disorders, arthritis, anxiety, depression and digestive concerns. Helps to promote general wellbeing.

AROMATHERAPY INDICATIONS

When we stretch the body we stretch the mind. Environmental Fragrancing is the ideal way to enhance your yoga practice, seducing the mind to surrender its control over matter. Remember if it matters in the mind, it 'matters' in the body. Use oils that have psychotherapeutic qualities. For the more enduring yoga styles such a Iyenga yoga, you may also wish to incorporate a body rub with essential oils to help your body relax and expand into each stretch. An Aromatic Bath revitalises tired muscles that have extended beyond the normal call of duty. Essential oils that optimise relaxation for extra stretch are Marjoram, Lavender, Orange, German and Roman Chamomile, Mandarin, Vetiver and Sandalwood.

Epilogue

A dear friend of ours, Glynn Braddy, told us a parable we thought perfect for the closing of this book:

"An old sage was sitting on the crest of a small hill. A woman approached him saying, 'Old man, I am with child. Teach me the ways of nature that I may bring this child forward in the highest expression of the Living Spirit. What must I eat, how much should I move, what personal disciplines and philosophy will serve this child that I may not diminish the natural beauty and power that is already within it? Tell me what I must know and I will do all that is required.'

And the old sage smiled. He gently brushed away the tear that had appeared on the mother's cheek and said, 'It has already been done.'"

If you should ever be overwhelmed by the options and opinions on the path to good health, remember your answer lies in the nature of your question.

Bibliography

Literature that we have scanned over the years helped us considerably in the compilation of this book.

We extend our thanks and appreciation to the authors of these books and journals.

Alexander, J. *Supertherapies*, Bantam Books, London, 1996.

Davis, P. *Aromatherapy An A-Z*, C.W. Daniel Company Limited, England, 1988.

Downes, K. & White J. *Aromatherapy for Scentual Awareness*, Nacson and Sons, Sydney 1992.

Shealy, C. N. *The Complete Guide To Alternative Medicine*, Element, Brisbane, 1996.

Kirchheimer, S. and the editors of Prevention Magazine *The doctors Book of Remedies II*, Bantam, New York, 1993.

Making The Right Choice

For effective therapeutic use, it is vital that only pure essential oils are used in aromatherapy. Do not fall into the trap of buying cheaper, impure oils. Often they do not work effectively on a therapeutic level and there may be bodily reactions to the additives.

Unscrupulous suppliers will sometimes dilute a pure essential oil in a massage base oil and pass it off as pure natural essence. For this reason, it is advisable that you purchase your oils from a reputable company.

Take Good Care

Not all plants and plant products are beneficial to health. Some are poisonous and dangerous. The authors encourage you to follow the guidelines in this book.

The material in this book is not meant to take the place of diagnosis and treatment by a qualified medical practitioner. The authors' recommendations in this book are based on their own experiences and their vast research. However, a small number of people may react differently to certain oils due to biochemical individuality.

For this reason, the authors make no guarantees as to the effects of their use and no liability will be accepted.

Discover More About Aromatherapy

Perhaps you would like to journey further into the scentual world of aromatherapy... Karen's and Judith's magazine, *Aromatherapy for Scents and Sensuality*, has sold over 250,000 copies internationally.

Other books by Karen and Judith include bestsellers *Aromatherapy for Scentual Awareness*, *Aromatherapy for Lovers and Dreamers* and *Aromatherapy for Men*.

Aromatherapy for Scentual Awareness is undoubtedly one of the most popular aromatherapy books in Australia. There are over 150,000 copies in print, and it is regarded by many as the ultimate introduction to aromatherapy.

Aromatherapy for Lovers and Dreamers, co-authored with Leon Nacson, explores the many ways aromatherapy can heighten the experience of some of life's greatest adventures including dreaming, daydreaming and loving.

Aromatherapy for Men highlights the use of essential oils for a man's unique personal needs. In this book men will learn a simple body care program to strengthen their vitality. Men can use these aromatic tools for success both professionally and intimately.

To be placed on our exclusive mailing list call + 61 3 9486 9688. Free call 1 800 802 036 or freefax 1 800 062 888.

For Additional Information

Acupuncture Association of Australia (AAcA)

Australian Acupuncture Association (AAcA)

Association of Massage Therapists (NSW)

Association of Remedial Masseurs (ARM)

Australian Association of Polarity Therapy (AAPT)

Australian Federation of Homoeopaths (AFH)

Australian Feldenkrais Guild

Australian Natural Therapists Association (ANTA)

Australian Osteopathic Association (AOA)

Australian Society of Alexander Technique (AUSTAT)

Australian Traditional Medicine Society (ATMS)

International Federation of Aromatherapists
(Australian Branch)

Reflexology Association of Australia

Reflexology Association of Australia (QLD)

Index

About the Authors

Judith White and Karen Downes are experienced Aromatherpists, health, beauty and lifestyle educators. They have both studied holistic aromatherapy in Europe the recognized centre of knowledge in this field. They have taught Aromatherapy to Doctors, Nurses, Natural Therapists, Beauty Therapists and run workshops and seminars lecturing to tens of thousands of people around the world, providing these people with the tools to transform their lives.

Their seminars and workshops were fun, practical and inspiring, giving participants many new perceptions and life skills. Today Judith resides in Australia and Karen in England and after more than two decades, they continue to uphold and share the daily self nurturing practices through the daily use of pure essential oils.

Their message is simple "You can magnify your health beauty and wellness through simple, daily, self nurturing practices infused with the power of aromatherapy "

For more information:

Contact Judith White on Judith@australianorganicbrands.com
And
Contact Karen Downes on .... karenleedownes@hotmail.com

www.ingramcontent.com/pod-product-compliance
Lightning Source LLC
Chambersburg PA
CBHW030322290526
45785CB00001B/467